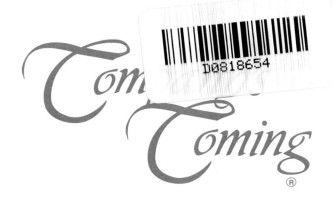

Low-Fat
Express

Jean Paré

www.companyscoming.com
visit our website

Back Cover

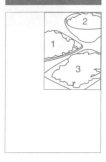

1. Mango Fennel Pork, page 68
2. Pork Bean Stew, page 70
3. Glazed Pork Chops, page 69

Props courtesy of: Danesco Inc.
The Bay
Winners Stores

We gratefully acknowledge the following suppliers for their generous support of our Test and Photography Kitchens:

Broil King Barbecues   *Hamilton Beach® Canada*   *Proctor Silex® Canada*
Corelle®   *Lagostina®*   *Tupperware®*

Low-Fat Express

Copyright © Company's Coming Publishing Limited

All rights reserved worldwide. No part of this book may be reproduced, stored in a retrieval system or transmitted in any form by any means without written permission in advance from the publisher.

In the case of photocopying or other reprographic copying, a license may be purchased from the Canadian Copyright Licensing Agency (Access Copyright). Visit www.accesscopyright.ca or call toll free 1-800-893-5777. In the United States, please contact the Copyright Clearance Centre at www.copyright.com or call 978-646-8600.

Brief portions of this book may be reproduced for review purposes, provided credit is given to the source. Reviewers are invited to contact the publisher for additional information.

First Printing March 2008

Library and Archives Canada Cataloguing in Publication
Paré, Jean, date-
Low-fat express / Jean Paré.
(Original series)
Includes index.
ISBN 978-1-897069-50-9
1. Low-fat diet—Recipes. I. Title. II. Series: Paré, Jean, date- . Original series.
RM237.7.P37 2008   641.5'6384   C2007-903930-8

Published by
Company's Coming Publishing Limited
2311 – 96 Street
Edmonton, Alberta, Canada T6N 1G3
Tel: 780-450-6223   Fax: 780-450-1857
www.companyscoming.com

Company's Coming is a registered trademark owned by
Company's Coming Publishing Limited

We acknowledge the financial support of the Government of Canada through the Book Publishing Industry Development Program (BPIDP) for our publishing activities.

Printed in China

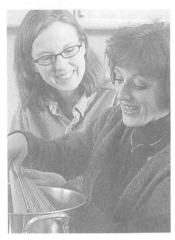

Need more recipes?

Six *"sneak preview"* recipes are featured online **with every new book released.**

Visit us at
www.companyscoming.com

Company's Coming Cookbooks

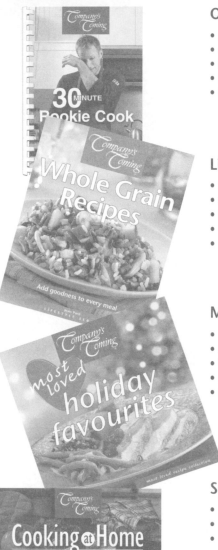

Original Series

- Softcover, 160 pages
- 6" x 9" (15 cm x 23 cm) format
- Lay-flat plastic comb binding
- Full-colour photos
- Nutrition information

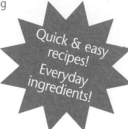

Quick & easy recipes! Everyday ingredients!

Lifestyle Series

- Softcover, 160 pages
- 8" x 10" (20 cm x 25 cm) format
- Paperback
- Full-colour photos
- Nutrition information

Most Loved Recipe Collection

- Hardcover, 128 pages
- 8 3/4" x 8 3/4" (22 cm x 22 cm) format
- Durable sewn binding
- Full-colour throughout
- Nutrition information

Special Occasion Series

- Hardcover concealed wiro
- 8 1/2" x 11" (22 cm x 28 cm) format
- Lay-flat binding
- Full-colour throughout
- Nutrition information

See page 157 for more cookbooks.
For a complete listing, visit
www.companyscoming.com

Table of Contents

The Company's Coming Story

Jean Paré (pronounced "jeen PAIR-ee") grew up understanding that the combination of family, friends and home cooking is the best recipe for a good life. From her mother, she learned to appreciate good cooking, while her father praised even her earliest attempts in the kitchen. When Jean left home, she took with her a love of cooking, many family recipes and an intriguing desire to read cookbooks as if they were novels!

"never share a recipe you wouldn't use yourself" In 1963, when her four children had all reached school age, Jean volunteered to cater the 50th Anniversary of the Vermilion School of Agriculture, now Lakeland College, in Alberta, Canada. Working out of her home, Jean prepared a dinner for more than 1,000 people, which launched a flourishing catering operation that continued for over 18 years. During that time, she had countless opportunities to test new ideas with immediate feedback—resulting in empty plates and contented customers! Whether preparing cocktail sandwiches for a house party or serving a hot meal for 1,500 people, Jean Paré earned a reputation for good food, courteous service and reasonable prices.

As requests for her recipes mounted, Jean was often asked the question, "Why don't you write a cookbook?" Jean responded by teaming up with her son, Grant Lovig, in the fall of 1980 to form Company's Coming Publishing Limited. The publication of *150 Delicious Squares* on April 14, 1981 marked the debut of what would soon become one of the world's most popular cookbook series.

The company has grown since those early days when Jean worked from a spare bedroom in her home. Today, she continues to write recipes while working closely with the staff of the Recipe Factory, as the Company's Coming test kitchen is affectionately known. There she fills the role of mentor, assisting with the development of recipes people most want to use for everyday cooking and easy entertaining. Every Company's Coming recipe is *kitchen-tested* before it's approved for publication.

Jean's daughter, Gail Lovig, is responsible for marketing and distribution, leading a team that includes sales personnel located in major cities across Canada. In addition, Company's Coming cookbooks are published and distributed under licence in the United States, Australia and other world markets. Bestsellers many times over in English, Company's Coming cookbooks have also been published in French and Spanish.

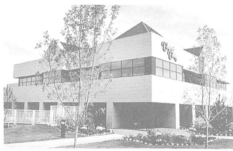

Familiar and trusted in home kitchens around the world, Company's Coming cookbooks are offered in a variety of formats. Highly regarded as kitchen workbooks, the softcover Original Series, with its lay-flat plastic comb binding, is still a favourite among readers.

Jean Paré's approach to cooking has always called for *quick and easy recipes* using *everyday ingredients*. That view has served her well. The recipient of many awards, including the Queen Elizabeth Golden Jubilee medal, Jean was appointed a Member of the Order of Canada, her country's highest lifetime achievement honour.

Jean continues to gain new supporters by adhering to what she calls The Golden Rule of Cooking: *"Never share a recipe you wouldn't use yourself."* It's an approach that works— *millions of times over!*

Foreword

We all know a diet of fast food and highly processed fare isn't the best way to feed our families. We've also heard about the increasing rates of obesity in our society and worry about our waistbands becoming increasingly tighter. But when life is jam-packed with work, meetings and piano lessons, not to mention the laundry, when are we supposed to cook something healthy?

If you've got 30 minutes, you can do it with *Low-Fat Express*. In the time it takes to order and wait for a less-than-healthy pizza to be delivered, you can pick any recipe from this book and prep it, cook it and put it on your table. The bonus? Each serving is less than 10 grams of fat.

From Chili Rubbed Steaks to Focaccia Pizza Pie, these delicious dinner ideas will satisfy every family member. You'll also find soups, salads and tasty appetizers, as well as great breakfasts and lunches.

Being mindful about what you eat doesn't mean you have to feel deprived. For snack attacks, we've created Oven Onion Rings and fabulous Cherry Macaroons. You'll also find desserts, such as Apples 'N' Maple Cream and a beautiful Peach Blueberry

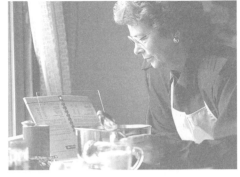

Cobbler—all of them under 10 grams of fat and all of them ready in half an hour.

How did we do it? For speed, we chose stove-top and grilling methods, as well as some convenience products, like lettuce mixes. For nutrition, we chose low-fat dairy products, leaner cuts of meat, egg products and more fresh ingredients. And when we did incorporate fats, we were choosy, opting for healthier varieties such as canola and olive oil or, in the case of baking, carefully considered amounts of butter.

Healthy isn't hard. All you need is 30 minutes and *Low-Fat Express*.

Jean Paré

Nutrition Information Guidelines

Each recipe is analyzed using the most current version of the Canadian Nutrient File from Health Canada, which is based on the United States Department of Agriculture (USDA) Nutrient Database.

- If more than one ingredient is listed (such as "butter or hard margarine"), or if a range is given (1 – 2 tsp., 5 – 10 mL), only the first ingredient or first amount is analyzed.

- For meat, poultry and fish, the serving size per person is based on the recommended 4 oz. (113 g) uncooked weight (without bone), which is 2 – 3 oz. (57 – 85 g) cooked weight (without bone)—approximately the size of a deck of playing cards.

- Milk used is 1% M.F. (milk fat), unless otherwise stated.

- Cooking oil used is canola oil, unless otherwise stated.

- Ingredients indicating "sprinkle," "optional," or "for garnish" are not included in the nutrition information.

- The fat in recipes and combination foods can vary greatly depending on the sources and types of fats used in each specific ingredient. For these reasons, the amount of saturated, monounsaturated and polyunsaturated fats may not add up to the total fat content.

Vera C. Mazurak, Ph.D.
Nutritionist

Getting factual about fat

The good, the bad and the ugly (fats)

Fat is not a four-letter word—in fact, medical scientists maintain that fat is an essential part of your daily diet. It helps you absorb fat-soluble vitamins, such as A, D, E and K, boosts your immune system and protects nerve cells. But you only need a small daily amount—two to three tablespoons or 30 to 45 mL—and some fats are better than others:

The good:
Monounsaturated and polyunsaturated fats raise your HDL or "good cholesterol" levels and lower your LDL or "bad cholesterol" levels. You can find these fats in avocados, fish, nuts, peanuts, seeds, canola and olive and sunflower oils, for example.

The bad:
Saturated fat and trans fatty acids (trans fat) are found in butter, hard margarine, meat, poultry, chocolate, lard and tropical oils such as coconut, palm kernel and palm. By raising blood levels of "bad cholesterol," these fats increase your risk of heart disease.

The ugly:
Though saturated fats raise your LDL cholesterol levels, they also have a small effect on raising your HDL levels. But trans fat *only* raises your LDL or "bad cholesterol" levels. While trans fat is found in small amounts in animal products, it's most common in manufactured food, such as hard margarine, crackers, cookies, pastries, muffins and fried foods, where it helps to lengthen shelf life. Since government regulations have made trans fat labelling mandatory on most foods, many manufacturers have moved away from using trans fat. If you can't find a nutrition label on the package, look for ingredients such as shortening, or hydrogenated or partially hydrogenated vegetable oil as an indication that the item includes trans fat. The absence of trans fat, however, doesn't mean that a food item is low-fat.

Fast fat facts

- Butter and regular margarine have the same amount of calories (100 per tbsp./15 mL).

- A tablespoon of butter has twice as many calories as a tablespoon of sugar.

- Eliminating fat won't eliminate calories, but it will eliminate high-calorie components in food.

- Losing weight or maintaining a healthy weight is not just about reducing dietary fat; it's also about portion control. Just because the dessert topping is low-fat, doesn't mean you can have five portions. (Well, you can, but all those calories have got to go somewhere…)

The condiment conundrum

Sometimes it really is the hidden fat that gets us. We order a salad for lunch, thinking we're doing great, but don't realize that the 3 tbsp. (50 mL) of regular ranch dressing just added 23 grams of fat and 220 calories to our "healthy" lunch. Be proactive when you're eating out and ask what low-fat condiments are available, because most restaurants, even fast food ones, offer them. Other condiments you may want to look out for are mayonnaise with 1 tbsp. (15 mL) weighing in with 11 grams of fat and 100 calories; and tartar sauce with 2 tbsp. (30 mL) packing in 7 grams of fat and 80 calories. But take heart, some of the best-loved condiments, like mustard, ketchup, relish and salsa, are pretty much fat-free.

Decoding the label lingo

It's easier to cut down on fat when we know where it's coming from. Let's look at a bag of tortilla chips, with a "Zero Trans Fats" banner on the front. The perfect, guilt-free snack? Not really. Let's have a closer look at the Nutrition Facts box on the back:

Nutrition Facts
Valeur nutritive
Per 11 chips (50 g)
par 11 croustilles (50 g)

Amount Teneur	% Daily Value % valeur quotidienne
Calories / Calories 260	
Fat / Lipides 13 g	20 %
Saturated / saturés 2 g	10 %
+ Trans / trans 0 g	
Cholesterol / Cholestérol 0 mg	0 %
Sodium / Sodium 340 mg	14 %
Carbohydrate / Glucides 32 g	11 %
Fibre / Fibres 2 g	7 %
Sugars / Sucres 2 g	
Protein / Protéines 3 g	
Vitamin A / Vitamine A	0 %
Vitamin C / Vitamine C	0 %
Calcium / Calcium	4 %
Iron / Fer	4 %

Serving size 11:
First shock: Only 11 chips—yes, 11—make up a serving, and they weigh 50 g, about the same as three cherry tomatoes.

Calories 260:
That means a single chip is worth 23.64 calories, about the same as eight cherry tomatoes.

Fat 13 g:
So if the serving size weighs 50 g, about one quarter of the 11 chips is made up of fat.

Fat 20%:
Most experts agree that an average person consuming 2,000 calories a day should have no more than 30 per cent, or 65 g, of those calories from fat. That's your daily fat allowance. With 11 of these chips, you've already eaten 20 per cent, or one/fifth of your daily fat allowance. Grab another handful or two, then sit down to a cheeseburger and French fries and you've blown your daily fat allowance. Guess where all that extra fat goes…

Trans 0 g:
As the bag says, these chips are made with zero trans fats. But right above it, you'll see 2 g of saturated fat, which is one of the fats to be avoided.

Sodium 14%:
Again, this is in only 11 chips. Doctors have warned patients for years about the link between too much salt and high blood pressure. They recommend a daily sodium limit of 2,400 mg, which equals about one teaspoon of salt. Sodium is an easy taste enhancer, but the herbs, spices and other flavourings used in *Low-Fat Express* make great alternatives.

Cutting the fat (right in the supermarket)

Cutting out calories—and fat—is easy, given the huge range of choices on grocery shelves these days. Consider some of these alternatives:

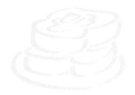

Higher-fat foods	Lower-fat foods
• Evaporated whole milk	• Evaporated skim or 2% milk
• Whole milk	• Skim, 1% or 2% milk
• Ice cream	• Sorbet, sherbet, low-fat frozen yogurt
• Sour cream	• Plain, low-fat yogurt
• Cream cheese	• Neufchatel or light cream cheese
• Mozzarella cheese	• Part-skim mozzarella cheese
• Ramen noodles	• Rice or pasta (spaghetti, fusilli, etc.)
• Granola	• Muesli
• Cold cuts or lunch meats	• Low-fat cold cuts
• Regular ground beef	• Lean ground beef
• Oil-packed tuna	• Water-packed tuna
• Frozen breaded or fried fish	• Fish fillets without breading
• Whole eggs	• Egg whites or substitutes
• Croissants, donuts, muffins, pastries	• English muffins, bagels, reduced-fat muffins
• Party crackers	• Soda or low-fat crackers
• Cookies	• Graham crackers, ginger snaps, fig bars
• Margarine or butter	• Light spread margarine or whipped butter*
• Mayonnaise and salad dressing	• Light versions
• Oil, shortening or lard	• Non-stick cooking spray for stir-frying or sautéing
• Toast topped with butter or margarine	• Toast topped with jam or honey

Note: These are not suitable alternatives for baking as they will change the outcome.

Mushroom Toasts

These crisp little toasts topped with creamy, rich mushrooms will get any party off to a dashingly delicious start. Best served hot.

Whole-wheat baguette bread slices (1/4 inch, 6 mm, thick)	16	16
Canola oil	2 tsp.	10 mL
Sliced fresh white mushrooms	3 cups	750 mL
Light herb and garlic cream cheese	2 tbsp.	30 mL
Light sour cream	1 tbsp.	15 mL
Pepper, sprinkle		

Preheat broiler. Arrange baguette slices in single layer on ungreased baking sheet. Broil on centre rack in oven for about 2 minutes per side until golden. Set aside.

Meanwhile, heat canola oil in large frying pan on medium. Add mushrooms. Cook for about 5 minutes, stirring occasionally, until browned and no liquid remains. Remove from heat.

Add remaining 3 ingredients. Stir until coated. Spoon mushroom mixture onto baguette slices. Makes 16 toasts.

1 toast: 31 Calories; 1.1 g Total Fat (0.3 g Mono, 0.2 g Poly, 0.3 g Sat); 2 mg Cholesterol; 4 g Carbohydrate; trace Fibre; 1 g Protein; 41 mg Sodium

Black Bean Fiesta Dip

This bean dip goes with everything from vegetable sticks to tortilla chips. Store leftovers in the fridge for up to five days.

Can of black beans, rinsed and drained	19 oz.	540 mL
Salsa	1/2 cup	125 mL
Non-fat plain yogurt	1/4 cup	60 mL
Chopped fresh cilantro or parsley	3 tbsp.	50 mL
Ground cumin	1/2 tsp.	2 mL

Put all 5 ingredients into blender or food processor. Process until smooth, scraping down sides if necessary. Makes about 2 cups (500 mL).

2 tbsp. (30 mL): 21 Calories; trace Total Fat (0 g Mono, trace Poly, 0 g Sat); trace Cholesterol; 5 g Carbohydrate; 2 g Fibre; 2 g Protein; 162 mg Sodium

Artichoke Lentil Dip

Make sure there are some healthy nibbles at your next get-together—this creamy, tangy, fat-free dip is perfect with raw veggies, low-fat crackers or toast points. Store in an airtight container in the fridge for up to one week.

Can of lentils, rinsed and drained	19 oz.	540 mL
Can of artichoke hearts, drained	14 oz.	398 mL
Fat-free sour cream	1 cup	250 mL
Sun-dried tomato pesto	2 tbsp.	30 mL
Pepper	1/4 tsp.	1 mL

Put all 5 ingredients into food processor. Process until smooth. Makes about 3 1/4 cups (800 mL).

1/4 cup (60 mL): 58 Calories; 0 g Total Fat (0 g Mono, 0 g Poly, 0 g Sat); 2 mg Cholesterol; 10 g Carbohydrate; 3 g Fibre; 4 g Protein; 173 mg Sodium

Goat Cheese Spread

There's a new cheese spread in town! Goat cheese with sweet bits of date adds a tangy twist to a favourite appetizer standby. Serve with low-fat crackers and celery sticks.

Soft goat (chèvre) cheese, softened	8 oz.	225 g
Skim milk	2 tbsp.	30 mL
Chopped pitted dates	1/2 cup	125 mL
Finely chopped fresh chives	2 tbsp.	30 mL
(or 1 1/2 tsp., 7 mL, dried)		
Balsamic vinegar	1 tbsp.	15 mL
Pepper	1/4 tsp.	1 mL

Mash cheese with fork in medium bowl. Add milk. Mix well.

Add remaining 4 ingredients. Stir well. Makes about 1 1/2 cups (375 mL).

2 tbsp. (30 mL): 71 Calories; 3.9 g Total Fat (0.9 g Mono, 0.1 g Poly, 2.7 g Sat); 8 mg Cholesterol; 6 g Carbohydrate; 1 g Fibre; 4 g Protein; 69 mg Sodium

Turkey Hoisin Rolls

We are firm believers in "hoisin" around the kitchen! Assemble these rolls yourself, or for a more casual get-together, just set out the turkey filling with the lettuce leaves and let your guests put their own together.

Canola oil	2 tsp.	10 mL
Chopped celery	1/2 cup	125 mL
Chopped onion	1/2 cup	125 mL
Finely grated gingerroot	2 tsp.	10 mL
(or 1/2 tsp., 2 mL, ground ginger)		
Garlic clove, minced	1	1
(or 1/4 tsp., 1 mL, powder)		
Extra-lean ground turkey	1/2 lb.	225 g
Finely chopped fresh white mushrooms	1/4 cup	60 mL
Hoisin sauce	2 tbsp.	30 mL
Chili paste (sambal oelek)	1/4 tsp.	1 mL
Finely chopped green onion	1/4 cup	60 mL
Butter lettuce leaves	32	32

Heat canola oil in large frying pan on medium. Add next 4 ingredients. Cook for about 5 minutes, stirring occasionally, until onion is softened.

Add turkey and mushrooms. Scramble-fry for about 5 minutes until turkey is no longer pink.

Add hoisin sauce and chili paste. Stir. Cook for about 4 minutes, stirring occasionally, until heated through.

Add green onion. Stir. Spoon about 1 tbsp. (15 mL) turkey mixture on each lettuce leaf. Roll to enclose filling. Makes 32 rolls.

1 roll: 16 Calories; 0.5 g Total Fat (0.2 g Mono, 0.1 g Poly, trace Sat); 3 mg Cholesterol; 1 g Carbohydrate; trace Fibre; 2 g Protein; 23 mg Sodium

Pictured on page 17.

Appetizers

Mustard Beef Crostini

These delightfully original appies of crisp toasts and tender beef topped with sweet honey Dijon sauce are sure to win rave reviews from your guests.

Beef top sirloin steak, trimmed of fat	3/4 lb.	340 g
Cooking spray		
Montreal steak spice	1/2 tsp.	2 mL
Fat-free sour cream	1/3 cup	75 mL
Dijon mustard	2 1/2 tbsp.	37 mL
Liquid honey	1 1/2 tsp.	7 mL
Baguette bread slices (1/4 inch, 6 mm, thick)	48	48
Cooking spray		

Preheat broiler. Spray both sides of steak with cooking spray. Sprinkle with steak spice. Place on greased broiler pan. Broil on top rack in oven for 3 to 5 minutes per side until desired doneness. Transfer to plate. Cover to keep warm.

Meanwhile, combine next 3 ingredients in small bowl.

Arrange baguette slices in single layer on ungreased baking sheet. Spray with cooking spray. Broil on top rack in oven for about 1 minute until golden. Cut steak into thin slices. Cut to fit baguette slices. Place 1 piece of steak on untoasted side of each baguette slice. Spoon about 1/2 tsp. (2 mL) mustard mixture over each steak slice. Makes 48 crostini.

1 crostini: 26 Calories; 0.6 g Total Fat (0.2 g Mono, trace Poly, 0.2 g Sat); 4 mg Cholesterol; 3 g Carbohydrate; trace Fibre; 2 g Protein; 49 mg Sodium

Pictured on page 17.

Chili Corn Crab Cakes

These mildly spicy, golden-brown cakes combine two favourites—corn fritters and crab cakes. With the added touch of sweet chili sauce, they're simply superb.

Large egg	1	1
Fine dry bread crumbs	6 tbsp.	100 mL
Sweet chili sauce	2 tbsp.	30 mL
Frozen kernel corn, thawed	1/2 cup	125 mL
Can of crabmeat, drained, cartilage removed, flaked	4 1/4 oz.	120 g
Finely diced celery	3 tbsp.	50 mL
Finely chopped green onion	2 tbsp.	30 mL
Salt	1/4 tsp.	1 mL
Pepper	1/4 tsp.	1 mL
Cooking Spray		

Preheat oven to 425°F (220°C). Beat egg with fork in medium bowl until frothy. Add bread crumbs and chili sauce. Mix well.

Add next 6 ingredients. Mix until mixture holds together in a ball. Divide into 8 equal portions. Shape into 1/2 inch (12 mm) thick cakes. Arrange on greased baking sheet. Spray cakes with cooking spray. Bake for about 10 minutes, turning at halftime, until golden. Serves 4.

1 serving: 107 Calories; 2.3 g Total Fat (0.9 g Mono, 0.4 g Poly, 0.6 g Sat); 73 mg Cholesterol; 11 g Carbohydrate; 1 g Fibre; 9 g Protein; 356 mg Sodium

Pictured at right.

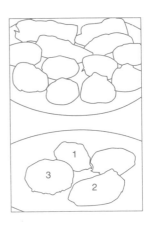

1. Turkey Hoisin Rolls, page 14
2. Mustard Beef Crostini, page 15
3. Chili Corn Crab Cakes, above

Props courtesy of: Mikasa Home Stores
Winners Stores

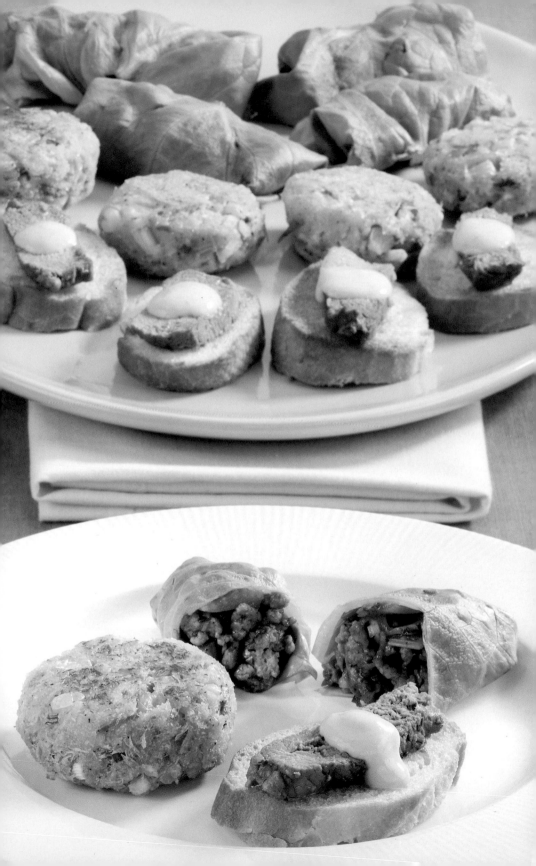

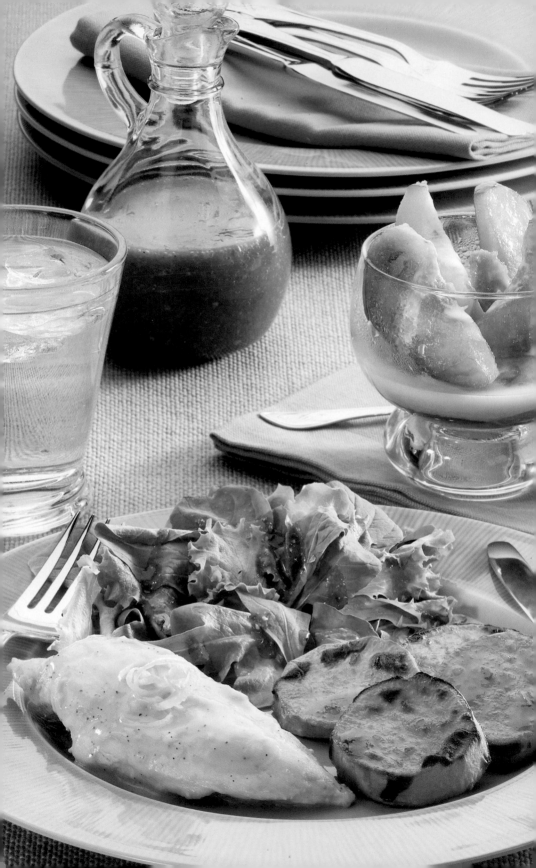

Creamy Mushroom Spread

Spread the word! This creamy spread combines tangy
balsamic vinegar with tender mushrooms and crunchy walnuts.
Great served on woven wheat crackers or toast points.

Butter (or hard margarine)	1 tsp.	5 mL
Chopped fresh white mushrooms	2 cups	500 mL
Finely diced onion	1/4 cup	60 mL
Balsamic vinegar	1 tsp.	5 mL
Garlic cloves, minced	1	1
(or 1/4 tsp., 1 mL, powder)		
Dried thyme	1/4 tsp.	1 mL
95% fat-free spreadable cream cheese	1/2 cup	125 mL
Chopped walnuts	1/4 cup	60 mL
Soy sauce	1 tsp.	5 mL
Worcestershire sauce	1 tsp.	5 mL
Pepper	1/4 tsp.	1 mL

Melt butter in medium frying pan on medium-high. Add next 5 ingredients.
Cook for about 5 minutes, stirring occasionally, until mushrooms are browned
and liquid is evaporated. Transfer to blender or food processor.

Add remaining 5 ingredients. Process until almost smooth. Makes about
1 cup (250 mL).

2 tbsp. (30 mL): 57 Calories; 3.1 g Total Fat (0.5 g Mono, 1.7 g Poly, 0.6 g Sat); 2 mg Cholesterol;
4 g Carbohydrate; trace Fibre; 4 g Protein; 122 mg Sodium

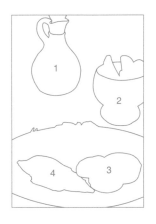

1. Roasted Red Pepper Dressing, page 56
2. Apples 'N' Maple Cream, page 134
3. Broiled Sweet Potatoes, page 118
4. Honey Dijon Lemon Chicken, page 79

Props courtesy of: Winners Stores

Tortillas With Corn Dip

These baked tortilla chips put store-bought ones to shame—and have a fraction of the fat! And the fabulously rich and tangy-sweet dip is the perfect complement.

TORTILLA WEDGES

Flour tortillas (7 1/2 inch, 19 cm, diameter)	4	4
Jalapeño jelly	3 tbsp.	50 mL
Ground cinnamon	1/2 tsp.	2 mL
Ground cumin	1/2 tsp.	2 mL

CORN DIP

95% fat-free spreadable cream cheese	1/2 cup	125 mL
Light sour cream	1/2 cup	125 mL
Corn relish	2 tbsp.	30 mL
Finely chopped pickled pepper rings	2 tbsp.	30 mL
Finely chopped canned sliced jalapeño pepper (see Tip, page 26)	1 tbsp.	15 mL
Salt	1/4 tsp.	1 mL
Pepper	1/4 tsp.	1 mL

Tortilla Wedges: Preheat oven to 350°F (175°C). Arrange tortillas on 2 baking sheets.

Combine next 3 ingredients in small cup. Brush jelly mixture evenly over tortillas. Cut tortillas into 8 wedges each. Bake on separate racks in oven for about 10 minutes, switching position of baking sheets at halftime, until crisp. Makes 32 wedges.

Corn Dip: Meanwhile, beat cream cheese and sour cream in small bowl until smooth.

Add remaining 5 ingredients. Stir well. Makes about 1 1/3 cups (325 mL) dip. Serve with tortilla wedges. Serves 8.

1 serving: 131 Calories; 3.4 g Total Fat (1.0 g Mono, 0.4 g Poly, 1.4 g Sat); 6 mg Cholesterol; 20 g Carbohydrate; 1 g Fibre; 5 g Protein; 332 mg Sodium

Appetizers

Creamy Black Bean Spirals

These easy-to-make spirals have a creamy and tangy filling
with just enough spicy kick to get the party started.

Block of light cream cheese, softened	4 oz.	125 g
Light sour cream	1/4 cup	60 mL
Salsa	2 tbsp.	30 mL
Canned black beans, rinsed and drained	1 cup	250 mL
Garlic powder	1/4 tsp.	1 mL
Chili powder	1/8 tsp.	0.5 mL
Flour tortillas (9 inch, 22 cm, diameter)	2	2

Beat cream cheese and sour cream in medium bowl until smooth. Stir in salsa. Set aside.

Put next 3 ingredients into food processor. Process until smooth.

Spread bean mixture on tortillas, almost to edge. Spread salsa mixture over top. Roll up tightly, jelly-roll style. Wrap with plastic wrap. Freeze for 15 minutes (see Note). Trim ends. Cut rolls into 1/2 inch (12 mm) slices. Makes about 32 spirals.

1 spiral: 22 Calories; 1.0 g Total Fat (0.2 g Mono, 0.1 g Poly, 0.5 g Sat); 2 mg Cholesterol;
3 g Carbohydrate; 1 g Fibre; 1 g Protein; 71 mg Sodium

Note: If you aren't going to serve these spirals right away, chill in the refrigerator instead of the freezer until you're ready to cut them.

Paré Pointer
Do shooting stars end up in jail?

Pepper Cheese Omelette

*This big baked omelette is filled with enough peppers, onions and cheese
to make a spectacular breakfast for you and someone special.*

Chopped red pepper	1/2 cup	125 mL
Chopped yellow (or green) pepper	1/2 cup	125 mL
Chopped onion	1/4 cup	60 mL
Salsa	2 tbsp.	30 mL
Large eggs (see Note)	2	2
Egg whites (large)	4	4
Salt, just a pinch		
Pepper, just a pinch		
Grated light sharp Cheddar cheese	1/4 cup	60 mL

Heat large frying pan on medium. Spray with cooking spray. Add first
3 ingredients. Cook for about 5 minutes, stirring occasionally, until onion
is softened. Transfer to small bowl.

Add salsa. Stir. Cover to keep warm.

Preheat broiler. Whisk next 4 ingredients in separate small bowl. Spray
same frying pan with cooking spray. Pour egg mixture into pan. Reduce
heat to medium-low. Cook, uncovered, for 2 to 4 minutes until bottom
is set. Broil on centre rack in oven (see Tip, below) for about 1 minute until
top is set and golden. Spoon salsa mixture over half of omelette.

Sprinkle cheese over salsa mixture. Fold omelette in half to cover cheese.
Serves 2.

*1 serving: 175 Calories; 7.6 g Total Fat (2.2 g Mono, 0.9 g Poly, 3.1 g Sat); 194 mg Cholesterol;
9 g Carbohydrate; 2 g Fibre; 19 g Protein; 329 mg Sodium*

Note: If cholesterol is a concern for you, replace the whole eggs and the
egg whites with egg product equivalent to 4 whole eggs.

 tip When baking or broiling food in a frying pan with a handle that isn't
ovenproof, wrap the handle in foil and keep it to the front of the oven,
away from the element.

Apple Raisin French Toast

*With a sweet apple cinnamon topping, this raisin
French toast is simply* magnifique!

APPLE CINNAMON TOPPING

Chopped peeled cooking apple (such as McIntosh)	1 cup	250 mL
Apple juice	2 tbsp.	30 mL
Brown sugar, packed	1 tbsp.	15 mL
Ground cinnamon	1/8 tsp.	0.5 mL

RAISIN FRENCH TOAST

Large egg	1	1
Egg whites (large)	2	2
Skim milk	1/4 cup	60 mL
Raisin bread slices	4	4

Apple Cinnamon Topping: Combine all 4 ingredients in small saucepan. Cover. Bring to a boil. Reduce heat to medium. Cook, uncovered, for about 5 minutes, stirring occasionally, until apple is tender. Makes about 1/2 cup (125 mL) topping.

Raisin French Toast: Meanwhile, whisk first 3 ingredients in small shallow bowl.

Dip 1 bread slice in egg mixture. Turn to coat both sides. Place on large plate. Repeat with remaining bread slices. Pour remaining egg mixture over top. Heat large frying pan on medium. Spray with cooking spray. Arrange bread slices in single layer in frying pan. Cook for about 2 minutes per side until browned. Transfer bread slices to 2 serving plates. Spoon Apple Cinnamon Topping over top. Serves 2.

1 serving: 271 Calories; 4.9 g Total Fat (2.3 g Mono, 0.8 g Poly, 1.4 g Sat); 94 mg Cholesterol; 46 g Carbohydrate; 4 g Fibre; 12 g Protein; 307 mg Sodium

Low-Fat Egg Muffins

These healthy whole-wheat egg muffins have the added attraction of tomato pesto to get your taste buds jumping.

Whole-wheat (or plain) English muffins, split	2	2
Butter	1 tbsp.	15 mL
Prepackaged egg white product	1 cup	250 mL
95% fat-free spreadable cream cheese	1/2 cup	125 mL
Skim milk	1/4 cup	60 mL
Sun-dried tomato pesto	2 tbsp.	30 mL
Chopped fresh parsley, sprinkle		
Paprika, sprinkle		

Toast English muffin halves. Cover to keep warm.

Meanwhile, melt butter in large frying pan on medium.

Whisk next 4 ingredients in medium bowl until combined. Pour into frying pan. Cook and stir until set and liquid is evaporated. Spoon over muffin halves.

Sprinkle with parsley and paprika. Serves 2.

1 serving: 312 Calories; 7.9 g Total Fat (2.0 g Mono, 0.8 g Poly, 4.4 g Sat); 20 mg Cholesterol; 33 g Carbohydrate; 5 g Fibre; 30 g Protein; 1142 mg Sodium

Apple Cinnamon Quinoa

When quinoa (pronounced KEEN-wah) is loaded with apples and cinnamon, it makes a breakfast that can't be beat.

Skim evaporated milk	1 cup	250 mL
Apple juice	1/2 cup	125 mL
Quinoa, rinsed and drained	1 cup	250 mL
Sweetened applesauce	1/2 cup	125 mL
Brown sugar, packed	2 tbsp.	30 mL
Ground cinnamon	1/2 tsp.	2 mL
Salt	1/8 tsp.	0.5 mL

(continued on next page)

Breakfasts

Combine milk and apple juice in large saucepan. Heat on medium until hot, but not boiling.

Add remaining 5 ingredients. Stir. Reduce heat to medium-low. Simmer, covered, for 20 to 25 minutes, stirring occasionally, until quinoa is tender. Makes about 2 2/3 cups (650 mL). Serves 4.

1 serving: 273 Calories; 2.7 g Total Fat (0.7 g Mono, 1.0 g Poly, 0.3 g Sat); 2 mg Cholesterol; 53 g Carbohydrate; 3 g Fibre; 10 g Protein; 161 mg Sodium

Apple Maple Cereal

Healthy needn't mean bland—with the addition of orange, apple and maple, plain old oatmeal becomes a delicious taste treat. Heat leftovers in the microwave with a little added orange juice.

Orange juice	1 1/2 cups	375 mL
Water	1/2 cup	125 mL
Bulgur	1/2 cup	125 mL
Large flake rolled oats	1/2 cup	125 mL
Medium peeled cooking apple (such as McIntosh), grated	1	1
Brown sugar, packed	2 tbsp.	30 mL
Maple (or maple-flavoured) syrup	2 tbsp.	30 mL
Ground cinnamon	1/2 tsp.	2 mL

Combine orange juice and water in medium saucepan. Bring to a boil. Reduce to medium-low. Add bulgur and oats. Stir. Cook, covered, for about 10 minutes, without stirring, until bulgur and oats are tender and liquid is absorbed.

Add remaining 4 ingredients. Stir. Let stand, covered, for 5 minutes. Makes about 3 cups (750 mL). Serves 4.

1 serving: 211 Calories; 1.2 g Total Fat (0.1 g Mono, 0.2 g Poly, 0.1 g Sat); 0 mg Cholesterol; 48 g Carbohydrate; 4 g Fibre; 5 g Protein; 8 mg Sodium

Calabacita Eggs

Put a little pep into your morning with this fresh and healthy concoction of veggies, eggs and cheese. Serve with a spicy salsa to put a little pep in your step.

Diced onion	1 cup	250 mL
Diced zucchini (with peel)	1 cup	250 mL
Diced red pepper	1/2 cup	125 mL
Diced jalapeño pepper (see Tip, below)	2 tbsp.	30 mL
Garlic powder	1/2 tsp.	2 mL
Salt	1/4 tsp.	1 mL
Frozen kernel corn, thawed	1 cup	250 mL
Chopped fresh cilantro or parsley (or 1 1/2 tsp., 7 mL, dried)	2 tbsp.	30 mL
Low-cholesterol egg product	1 1/2 cups	375 mL
Pepper	1/4 tsp.	1 mL
Grated light sharp Cheddar cheese	1/2 cup	125 mL

Heat large frying pan on medium. Spray with cooking spray. Add onion. Cook for about 5 minutes, stirring often, until onion starts to soften.

Add next 5 ingredients. Cook for about 5 minutes, stirring occasionally, until zucchini is tender-crisp.

Add corn and cilantro. Cook and stir for about 1 minute until heated through.

Meanwhile, beat egg product and pepper with fork in medium bowl. Pour over vegetable mixture. Cook and stir for about 2 minutes until set.

Sprinkle cheese over top. Remove from heat. Let stand, covered, for about 1 minute until cheese is melted. Makes about 5 cups (1.25 L). Serves 4.

1 serving: 155 Calories; 4.3 g Total Fat (trace Mono, 0.1 g Poly, 1.5 g Sat); 85 mg Cholesterol; 15 g Carbohydrate; 2 g Fibre; 14 g Protein; 368 mg Sodium

Pictured on page 35.

 tip   Hot peppers contain capsaicin in the seeds and ribs. Removing the seeds and ribs will reduce the heat. Wear rubber gloves when handling hot peppers and avoid touching your eyes. Wash your hands well afterwards.

Orange Chai Muffins

Mild orange and exotic chai flavours infuse these tender,
moist muffins with a hip coffee house taste. Best served warm.

All-purpose flour	1 1/2 cups	375 mL
Quick-cooking rolled oats (not instant)	1 cup	250 mL
Baking powder	2 tsp.	10 mL
Baking soda	1/2 tsp.	2 mL
Salt	1/2 tsp.	2 mL
Large eggs	2	2
Sweetened chai tea concentrate	3/4 cup	175 mL
Brown sugar, packed	1/3 cup	75 mL
Orange juice	1/4 cup	60 mL
Canola oil	3 tbsp.	50 mL
Grated orange zest	1 tsp.	5 mL
Vanilla extract	1 tsp.	5 mL

Preheat oven to 400°F (205°C). Measure first 5 ingredients into large bowl. Stir. Make a well in centre.

Whisk remaining 7 ingredients in medium bowl. Add to well. Stir until just moistened. Fill 24 greased mini-muffin cups full. Bake for about 12 minutes until wooden pick inserted in centre of muffin comes out clean. Let stand in pan for 5 minutes. Remove muffins from pan and place on wire rack to cool. Makes 24 mini-muffins.

1 mini-muffin: 74 Calories; 2.4 g Total Fat (1.2 g Mono, 0.6 g Poly, 0.3 g Sat); 16 mg Cholesterol; 11 g Carbohydrate; 1 g Fibre; 2 g Protein; 103 mg Sodium

Pictured on page 35.

Orange Granola

Crispy orange-and-cinnamon flavoured oats with toasted almonds, coconut and sweet apricots make the perfect breakfast cereal—whether over yogurt or drenched in milk. Keep extras in the fridge for up to two weeks.

Liquid honey	1/4 cup	60 mL
Frozen concentrated orange juice	2 tbsp.	30 mL
Vanilla extract	1 tbsp.	15 mL
Canola oil	2 tsp.	10 mL
Ground cinnamon	1 tsp.	5 mL
Grated orange zest (optional)	1 tsp.	5 mL
Large flake rolled oats	3 cups	750 mL
Finely chopped dried apricot	1/2 cup	125 mL
Medium sweetened coconut	1/4 cup	60 mL
Sliced natural almonds	1/4 cup	60 mL

Preheat oven to 375°F (190°C). Combine first 6 ingredients in small dish. Reserve 2 tbsp. (30 mL) in small cup. Set aside.

Put oats into medium bowl. Drizzle remaining honey mixture over top. Stir until coated. Spread evenly on greased baking sheet with sides. Bake for about 5 minutes, stirring occasionally, until starting to crisp and lightly brown.

Meanwhile, combine remaining 3 ingredients in small bowl. Drizzle reserved honey mixture over top. Stir until coated. Add to oat mixture. Stir. Bake for 4 to 6 minutes until crisp and golden. Transfer baking sheet to wire rack to cool. Makes about 4 cups (1 L). Serves 8.

1 serving: 232 Calories; 5.8 g Total Fat (2.0 g Mono, 0.8 g Poly, 0.9 g Sat); 0 mg Cholesterol; 38 g Carbohydrate; 4 g Fibre; 7 g Protein; 12 mg Sodium

Pictured on page 35.

Maple Turkey Patties

A great alternative to regular breakfast sausage, these healthy turkey patties with a hint of sweet raisin flavour are great to wake up to.

Raisin bread slices	3	3
Large egg, fork-beaten	1	1
Grated peeled cooking apple (such as McIntosh)	1/2 cup	125 mL
Maple (or maple-flavoured) syrup	2 tbsp.	30 mL
Seasoned salt	1 tsp.	5 mL
Ground cinnamon	1/2 tsp.	2 mL
Poultry seasoning	1/2 tsp.	2 mL
Extra-lean ground turkey breast	1 lb.	454 g

Put bread slices into blender. Process until broken up into small pieces.

Preheat broiler. Combine next 6 ingredients and bread crumbs in medium bowl.

Add turkey. Mix well. Divide into 12 equal portions. Shape into 2 1/2 inch (6.4 cm) diameter patties. Arrange on greased baking sheet with sides. Broil on top rack in oven for about 5 minutes per side until browned and internal temperature reaches 175°F (80°C). Serves 6.

1 serving: 151 Calories; 2.4 g Total Fat (0.7 g Mono, 0.2 g Poly, 0.4 g Sat); 61 mg Cholesterol; 13 g Carbohydrate; 1 g Fibre; 21 g Protein; 338 mg Sodium

Paré Pointer

Nobody notices when you do the housework, but they sure notice when you don't.

Lemon Melon Berries

Fresh fruit salad with a light lemon mint syrup is bound
to make the best of anyone's a.m. Or serve with frozen
yogurt or light whipped topping for a healthy dessert.

Granulated sugar	1/3 cup	75 mL
Water	1/3 cup	75 mL
Grated lemon zest (see Tip, below)	1 tbsp.	15 mL
Lemon juice	2 tbsp.	30 mL
Cubed cantaloupe (or honeydew)	3 cups	750 mL
Sliced fresh strawberries	2 cups	500 mL
Fresh blueberries	1 cup	250 mL
Fresh raspberries (or blackberries), optional	1 cup	250 mL
Chopped fresh mint	2 tsp.	10 mL

Combine first 3 ingredients in small saucepan. Bring to a boil. Reduce heat to medium. Boil gently, uncovered, for about 5 minutes, stirring occasionally, until liquid is a thin syrup consistency. Remove from heat.

Add lemon juice. Stir. Let stand for about 5 minutes until slightly cooled.

Meanwhile, put next 4 ingredients into large bowl. Pour lemon mixture over fruit.

Sprinkle with mint. Toss. Serve immediately. Makes about 6 cups (1.5 L). Serves 6.

1 serving: 102 Calories; 0.4 g Total Fat (trace Mono, 0.2 g Poly, 0.1 g Sat); 0 mg Cholesterol; 26 g Carbohydrate; 3 g Fibre; 1 g Protein; 14 mg Sodium

Pictured on page 35.

 tip When a recipe calls for grated lemon zest and juice, it's easier to grate the lemon first, then juice it. Be careful not to grate down to the pith (white part of the peel), which is bitter and best avoided.

Sesame Chicken Pitas

The nutty taste of sesame is heightened by brown sugar and orange flavours.
Grab a napkin or two—these are magnificently messy!

Orange juice	3 tbsp.	50 mL
Light mayonnaise	1 tbsp.	15 mL
Sesame oil (for flavour)	1 tbsp.	15 mL
Brown sugar, packed	2 tsp.	10 mL
Finely grated gingerroot	2 tsp.	10 mL
(or 1/2 tsp., 2 mL, ground ginger)		
Soy sauce	1 tsp.	5 mL
Canola oil	1 tsp.	5 mL
Boneless, skinless chicken breast halves,	1/2 lb.	225 g
cut into 1/2 inch (12 mm) strips		
Cut or torn leaf lettuce (or spinach leaves),	2 cups	500 mL
lightly packed		
Whole-wheat pita breads	2	2
(7 inch, 18 cm, diameter),		
halved and opened		
Can of mandarin orange segments, drained	10 oz.	284 mL
Sliced red onion	1/4 cup	60 mL
Sesame seeds	1 tbsp.	15 mL

Combine first 6 ingredients in small cup. Set aside.

Heat large frying pan on medium-high until very hot. Add canola oil. Add chicken. Stir-fry for about 5 minutes until no longer pink inside. Transfer to small bowl. Cover to keep warm.

Put lettuce into medium bowl. Pour half of orange juice mixture over top. Toss. Spoon into pita pockets.

Add remaining 3 ingredients to chicken. Add remaining orange juice mixture. Toss gently. Spoon into pita pockets. Serves 4.

1 serving: 282 Calories; 8.8 g Total Fat (3.4 g Mono, 3.3 g Poly, 1.1 g Sat); 34 mg Cholesterol; 34 g Carbohydrate; 4 g Fibre; 19 g Protein; 333 mg Sodium

Toasted Tuna Sandwiches

*"Chicken of the sea" becomes the king of the sandwiches with
low-fat cheese and diced veggies. Smart food for sure!*

Cans of chunk light tuna in water (6 oz., 170 g, each), drained	2	2
Grated light Havarti cheese	3/4 cup	175 mL
95% fat-free spreadable cream cheese	1/4 cup	60 mL
Finely chopped dill pickle	2 tbsp.	30 mL
Finely diced celery	2 tbsp.	30 mL
Finely diced red pepper	2 tbsp.	30 mL
Sweet pickle relish	2 tbsp.	30 mL
Pepper	1/4 tsp.	1 mL
Whole-wheat Texas bread slices, toasted	4	4

Combine first 8 ingredients in medium bowl.

Preheat broiler. Arrange toast on baking sheet with sides. Spread tuna mixture evenly over each toast. Broil on centre rack in oven for about 5 minutes until heated through. Serves 4.

1 serving: 454 Calories; 10.0 g Total Fat (0.9 g Mono, 0.5 g Poly, 5.1 g Sat); 71 mg Cholesterol; 49 g Carbohydrate; 4 g Fibre; 42 g Protein; 1609 mg Sodium

Chicken Chutney Pizza

*Mango chutney gives this chicken pizza its uniquely Indian inspiration.
Add the South Seas sweetness of pineapple and lunch is a pleasure.*

Prebaked pizza crust (12 inch, 30 cm, diameter)	1	1
Mango chutney, larger pieces chopped	1/2 cup	125 mL
Chopped cooked chicken breast (see Tip, page 50)	1 cup	250 mL
Chopped green pepper	1/4 cup	60 mL
Chopped red pepper	1/2 cup	125 mL
Canned pineapple tidbits, drained	1/2 cup	125 mL
Grated part-skim mozzarella cheese	1/2 cup	125 mL

(continued on next page)

Lunches

Preheat oven to 475°F (240°C). Place crust on 12 inch (30 cm) pizza pan. Spread chutney evenly over crust.

Sprinkle remaining 5 ingredients, in order given, over chutney. Bake on bottom rack in oven for about 10 minutes until crust is browned. Cuts into 8 wedges. Serves 4.

1 serving: 284 Calories; 9.8 g Total Fat (2.3 g Mono, 1.8 g Poly, 1.9 g Sat); 33 mg Cholesterol; 26 g Carbohydrate; 1 g Fibre; 22 g Protein; 538 mg Sodium

---

BBQ Steak Wrap

Wrap up this meaty masterpiece, slather it with sauce and toss in some onions and tomatoes for a superb mid-day break.

Beef top sirloin steak, trimmed of fat	3/4 lb.	340 g
Seasoned salt	1/8 tsp.	0.5 mL
Pepper	1/8 tsp.	0.5 mL
Roma (plum) tomatoes, halved lengthwise	2	2
Red onion slices (1/2 inch,12 mm, thick)	4	4
Barbecue sauce	2 tbsp.	30 mL
Flour tortillas (9 inch, 22 cm, diameter)	4	4
Cut or torn romaine lettuce, lightly packed	3 cups	750 mL

Preheat gas barbecue to medium-high. Sprinkle steak with seasoned salt and pepper. Arrange steak, tomato and onion on greased grill.

Brush steak with barbecue sauce. Close lid. Cook steak for 2 to 4 minutes per side, brushing with barbecue sauce, until desired doneness. Transfer to cutting board. Cover to keep warm. Cook tomato and onion for 5 to 8 minutes, turning once, until softened and grill marks appear. Slice steak. Chop onion and tomato.

Meanwhile, wrap tortillas in foil. Heat on upper rack of gas barbecue for about 5 minutes, turning at halftime. Arrange steak slices along centre of tortillas.

Arrange lettuce over steak. Sprinkle tomato mixture over top. Fold in sides. Roll up from bottom to enclose filling. Serves 4.

1 serving: 272 Calories; 9.7 g Total Fat (2.5 g Mono, 0.4 g Poly, 3.2 g Sat); 45 mg Cholesterol; 24 g Carbohydrate; 2 g Fibre; 22 g Protein; 410 mg Sodium

Prosciutto Pear Panini

"Pearing" goat cheese and prosciutto with honey Dijon
is a delightful deal—a hearty gourmet lunch on the go!

Whole-grain (or white) baguette bread loaf, halved lengthwise	1	1
Cooking spray		
Soft goat (chèvre) cheese, softened	4 1/2 oz.	125 g
Dried thyme	1/4 tsp.	1 mL
Shredded green leaf lettuce, lightly packed	1 cup	250 mL
Thinly sliced prosciutto (or deli) ham	4 oz.	113 g
Large unpeeled pear, thinly sliced	1	1
Honey Dijon mustard	2 tbsp.	30 mL
Pepper	1/4 tsp.	1 mL

Preheat broiler. Place baguette halves, cut-side up, on baking sheet. Spray with cooking spray. Broil on top rack in oven for about 1 minute until lightly browned.

Spread goat cheese on bottom half of loaf. Sprinkle with thyme. Layer next 3 ingredients, in order given, over thyme.

Spread mustard on top half of loaf. Sprinkle with pepper. Place, mustard-side down, over pear. Press down lightly. Cuts into 6 pieces. Serves 6.

1 serving: 219 Calories; 7.9 g Total Fat (1.0 g Mono, 0.1 g Poly, 3.8 g Sat); 25 mg Cholesterol; 27 g Carbohydrate; 4 g Fibre; 14 g Protein; 852 mg Sodium

Pictured on page 36.

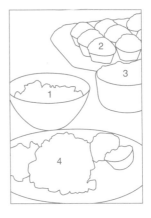

1. Orange Granola, page 28
2. Orange Chai Muffins, page 27
3. Lemon Melon Berries, page 30
4. Calabacita Eggs, page 26

Props courtesy of: Casa Bugatti
Winners Stores

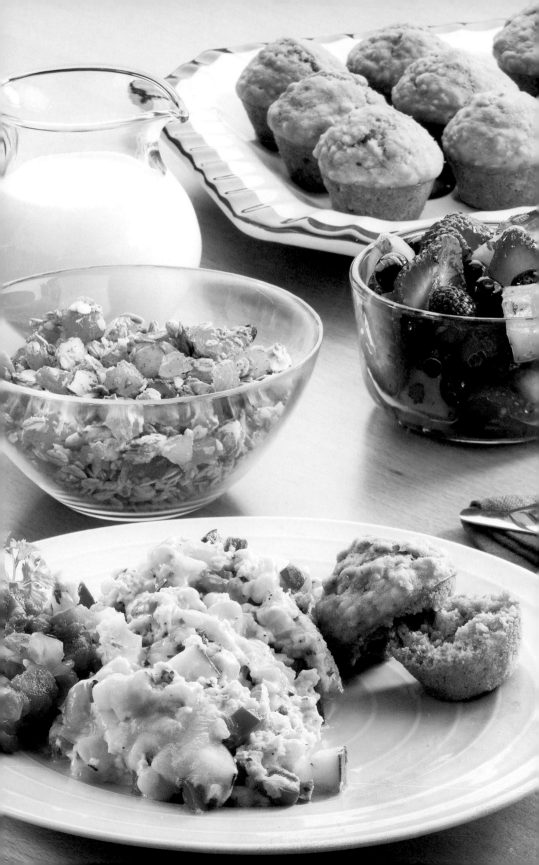

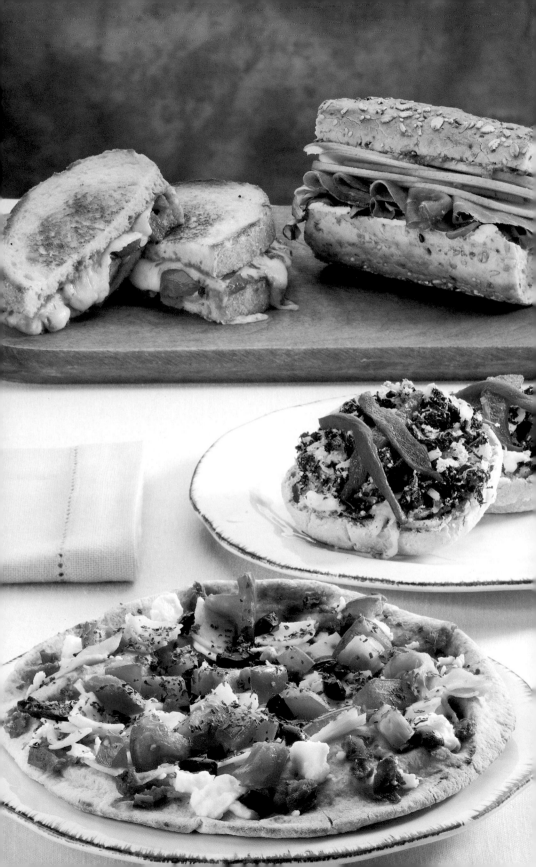

Grilled Basil Tomato Sandwich

Fresh tomatoes and basil give this sandwich a classic bruschetta flair.
Go ahead—get a little saucy for lunch.

Pizza sauce	2 tbsp.	30 mL
Italian (or French) bread slices	4	4
Grated part-skim mozzarella cheese	2/3 cup	150 mL
Chopped tomato	1/4 cup	60 mL
Roasted red peppers, blotted dry and chopped	1/4 cup	60 mL
Chopped fresh basil	1 tbsp.	15 mL
Cooking spray		

Spread pizza sauce on 1 side of each bread slice. Sprinkle cheese over sauce. Press down lightly.

Combine next 3 ingredients in small bowl. Spread over cheese on 2 bread slices. Place remaining bread slices, cheese-side down, over tomato mixture.

Heat large frying pan on medium. Spray both sides of sandwiches lightly with cooking spray. Place sandwiches in pan. Cook for about 2 minutes until bottoms are golden. Turn sandwiches over. Press down with spatula. Cook for another 2 minutes until bottoms are golden and cheese is melted. Serves 2.

1 serving: 335 Calories; 10.0 g Total Fat (2.9 g Mono, 0.7 g Poly, 5.1 g Sat); 26 mg Cholesterol; 42 g Carbohydrate; 4 g Fibre; 18 g Protein; 812 mg Sodium

Pictured at left.

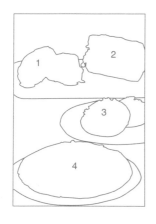

1. Grilled Basil Tomato Sandwhich, above
2. Prosciutto Pear Panini, page 34
3. Spinach Feta Melts, page 39
4. Pesto Pita Pizzas, page 38

Props courtesy of: Pier 1 Imports

Smoked Turkey Sandwich

A sandwich with a southwestern flare! Take smoked turkey and corn relish, add that creamy dressing and you're ready for lunch on the patio or packed in a picnic basket.

Chopped celery	1/2 cup	125 mL
Corn relish	1/2 cup	125 mL
Fat-free ranch dressing	1/4 cup	60 mL
Chopped roasted red pepper, blotted dry	2 tbsp.	30 mL
Onion buns, split	4	4
Deli smoked turkey slices	8 oz.	225 g
Tomato slices	8	8

Combine first 4 ingredients in small bowl.

Spread relish mixture on cut sides of buns. Serve turkey and tomato slices in buns. Serves 4.

1 serving: 288 Calories; 3.4 g Total Fat (trace Mono, 0.1 g Poly, 1.1 g Sat); 25 mg Cholesterol; 43 g Carbohydrate; 2 g Fibre; 20 g Protein; 892 mg Sodium

Pesto Pita Pizzas

Simple in a snap! Pesto and olives give these pita pizzas their pizzazz, and turkey gives them their protein. Fit for the whole family.

Pita breads (7 inch, 18 cm, diameter)	4	4
Sun-dried tomato pesto	8 tsp.	40 mL
Crumbled light feta cheese	1 cup	250 mL
Chopped deli turkey breast slices	1 cup	250 mL
Chopped kalamata olives	1/4 cup	60 mL
Chopped tomato	1 cup	250 mL
Dried basil	2 tsp.	10 mL

Preheat oven to 400°F (205°C). Arrange pitas on 2 baking sheets. Spread 2 tsp. (10 mL) pesto on each pita. Layer next 4 ingredients, in order given, over pesto.

(continued on next page)

Sprinkle basil over top. Bake on separate racks in oven for about 10 minutes, switching position of baking sheets at halftime, until pitas are crisp and cheese is melted. Serves 4.

1 serving: 349 Calories; 8.4 g Total Fat (0.8 g Mono, 0.5 g Poly, 4.3 g Sat); 46 mg Cholesterol; 42 g Carbohydrate; 2 g Fibre; 30 g Protein; 1853 mg Sodium

Pictured on page 36.

Spinach Feta Melts

Spinach is not only healthy, but tastes great in this tasty cheesy melt. Easy to make and packed with mega flavour!

Large egg	1	1
Box of frozen chopped spinach, thawed and squeezed dry	10 oz.	300 g
Crumbled light feta cheese	1/2 cup	125 mL
Grated part-skim mozzarella cheese	1/2 cup	125 mL
Fine dry bread crumbs	3 tbsp.	50 mL
Dried dillweed	1/2 tsp.	2 mL
Dried oregano	1/2 tsp.	2 mL
Garlic powder	1/4 tsp.	1 mL
Pepper	1/4 tsp.	1 mL
Whole-wheat (or plain) English muffins, split	4	4
Roasted red peppers, blotted dry and cut into 1/4 inch (6 mm) strips	1/4 cup	60 mL

Preheat oven to 350°F (175°C). Beat egg with fork in medium bowl until frothy. Add next 8 ingredients. Mix well.

Arrange muffin halves, cut-side up, on ungreased baking sheet with sides. Spread spinach mixture on muffin halves. Arrange red pepper strips over top. Bake for about 20 minutes until cheese is lightly golden. Serves 4.

1 serving: 286 Calories; 8.8 g Total Fat (1.6 g Mono, 0.9 g Poly, 4.4 g Sat); 67 mg Cholesterol; 35 g Carbohydrate; 6 g Fibre; 20 g Protein; 838 mg Sodium

Pictured on page 36.

Fettuccine Alfredo

Who would have thought a low-fat version of a classic favourite would be so tasty? You can have all that flavour without the added calories going to your waistline.

Water	12 cups	3 L
Salt	1 1/2 tsp.	7 mL
Fettuccine	8 oz.	225 g
1% milk	1/2 cup	125 mL
All-purpose flour	2 tbsp.	30 mL
Can of 2% evaporated milk	13 1/2 oz.	385 mL
95% fat-free spreadable cream cheese	2 tbsp.	30 mL
Garlic powder	1/4 tsp.	1 mL
Ground nutmeg	1/4 tsp.	1 mL
Salt	1/4 tsp.	1 mL
Pepper	1/4 tsp.	1 mL

Combine water and first amount of salt in Dutch oven or large pot. Bring to a boil. Add fettuccine. Boil, uncovered, for 11 to 13 minutes, stirring occasionally, until tender but firm. Drain. Return to same pot. Cover to keep warm.

Meanwhile, whisk milk into flour in small bowl until smooth.

Combine remaining 6 ingredients in medium saucepan. Heat and stir on medium until cream cheese is melted. Slowly add flour mixture, stirring constantly with whisk, until smooth. Heat and stir until boiling and slightly thickened. Add fettuccine. Toss until coated. Makes about 5 cups (1.25 L). Serves 4.

1 serving: 329 Calories; 3.2 g Total Fat (0.8 g Mono, 0.1 g Poly, 1.7 g Sat); 10 mg Cholesterol; 58 g Carbohydrate; 2 g Fibre; 17 g Protein; 311 mg Sodium

Variation: Use 2 tbsp. (30 mL) roasted garlic cream cheese instead of plain cream cheese and garlic powder.

Chili Macaroni And Cheese

No need to worry about the fat in this standby staple. Our mac 'n' cheese is given a new twist with tangy green chilis. It'll put a kick into your lunchtime.

Water	8 cups	2 L
Salt	1 tsp.	5 mL
Elbow macaroni	3 cups	750 mL
Skim milk	1 1/2 cups	375 mL
All-purpose flour	2 tbsp.	30 mL
Grated light sharp Cheddar cheese	1 1/2 cups	375 mL
95% fat-free spreadable cream cheese	1/2 cup	125 mL
Can of diced green chilies	4 oz.	113 g
Garlic powder	1/4 tsp.	1 mL
Salt	1/2 tsp.	2 mL
Pepper	1/4 tsp.	1 mL

Combine water and first amount of salt in Dutch oven. Bring to a boil. Add macaroni. Boil, uncovered, for 8 to 10 minutes, stirring occasionally, until tender but firm. Drain. Return to same pot. Cover to keep warm.

Meanwhile, whisk milk into flour in medium saucepan until smooth. Heat and stir on medium for 5 to 10 minutes until boiling and thickened.

Add Cheddar and cream cheese. Heat and stir until melted and smooth.

Add remaining 4 ingredients. Stir. Pour over macaroni. Stir until coated. Makes about 6 1/2 cups (1.6 L). Serves 4.

1 serving: 475 Calories; 8.6 g Total Fat (0.3 g Mono, 0.5 g Poly, 5.0 g Sat); 26 mg Cholesterol; 70 g Carbohydrate; 2 g Fibre; 30 g Protein; 793 mg Sodium

Cheesy Enchiladas

*A rainbow of colour and south-of-the-border tastes are abundant
in our cheesy enchiladas with salsa sauce. Pretty enough to eat!*

95% fat-free spreadable cream cheese	1/2 cup	125 mL
Light sour cream	1/2 cup	125 mL
Taco seasoning mix (stir before measuring)	1/2 tsp.	2 mL
Sliced green onion	2 tbsp.	30 mL
Flour tortillas (7 1/2 inch, 19 cm, diameter)	6	6
Salsa	1 cup	250 mL
Grated light sharp Cheddar cheese	1 cup	250 mL
Taco seasoning mix (stir before measuring)	1/2 tsp.	2 mL

Preheat oven to 425°F (220°C). Beat first 3 ingredients in medium bowl
until smooth. Add green onion. Stir well.

Spoon about 3 tbsp. (50 mL) cream cheese mixture along centre
of each tortilla. Fold in sides. Roll up from bottom to enclose filling.
Place, seam-side down, in greased 2 quart (2 L) shallow baking dish.

Pour salsa over tortillas. Sprinkle with cheese. Sprinkle with second
amount of taco seasoning. Bake for 15 to 20 minutes until Cheddar
cheese is melted and bubbling. Serves 6.

*1 serving: 235 Calories; 9.0 g Total Fat (0.1 g Mono, 0.1 g Poly, 4.2 g Sat); 18 mg Cholesterol;
27 g Carbohydrate; 1 g Fibre; 13 g Protein; 774 mg Sodium*

Paré Pointer
Forbidden fruit always makes bad jam.

Lunches

Gingered Pumpkin Soup

Pump(kin) up the flavour volume with this comforting, creamy soup
with the delicate tastes of ginger and orange.

Olive (or canola) oil	2 tsp.	10 mL
Chopped onion	1/2 cup	125 mL
Finely grated gingerroot	1 tbsp.	15 mL
(or 1/2 tsp., 2 mL, ground ginger)		
Garlic clove, minced	1	1
(or 1/4 tsp., 1 mL, powder)		
Ground nutmeg	1/2 tsp.	2 mL
Prepared chicken broth	2 cups	500 mL
Can of pure pumpkin (no spices)	14 oz.	398 mL
Orange juice	1 cup	250 mL
Brown sugar, packed	1 tbsp.	15 mL
Salted, roasted shelled pumpkin seeds	2 tbsp.	30 mL

Heat olive oil in large saucepan on medium. Add onion. Cook, uncovered, for about 5 minutes, stirring often, until softened.

Add next 3 ingredients. Stir. Cook for about 1 minute until fragrant.

Add next 4 ingredients. Stir. Simmer, uncovered, for 5 minutes, stirring occasionally, to blend flavours. Carefully process with hand blender or in blender until smooth.

Sprinkle pumpkin seeds over top. Makes about 4 cups (1 L). Serves 4.

1 serving: 126 Calories; 3.8 g Total Fat (2.1 g Mono, 0.6 g Poly, 0.8 g Sat); 0 mg Cholesterol; 22 g Carbohydrate; 3 g Fibre; 3 g Protein; 761 mg Sodium

Asian Meatball Soup

Meatballs may be unexpected in an Asian-style soup, but they're
absolutely at home in this light and delicate ginger and soy broth.

MEATBALLS

Large egg, fork-beaten	1	1
Fine dry bread crumbs	3 tbsp.	50 mL
Finely chopped water chestnut	2 tbsp.	30 mL
Soy sauce	2 tsp.	10 mL
Cornstarch	1 tsp.	5 mL
Finely grated gingerroot	1 tsp.	5 mL
(or 1/4 tsp., 1 mL, powder)		
Salt	1/4 tsp.	1 mL
Pepper	1/4 tsp.	1 mL
Extra-lean ground chicken (breast)	6 oz.	170 g
Frozen, uncooked shrimp	1 oz.	28 g
(peeled and deveined),		
thawed and finely chopped		

SOUP

Low-sodium prepared chicken broth	6 cups	1.5 L
Gingerroot slices (1/4 inch, 6 mm, thick)	3	3
Medium rice stick noodles, broken into	4 oz.	113 g
2 inch (5 cm) pieces		
Thinly sliced bok choy	2 cups	500 mL
Chopped green onion	1	1

Meatballs: Combine first 8 ingredients in medium bowl.

Add chicken and shrimp. Mix well. Roll into 3/4 inch (2 cm) balls.

Soup: Combine broth and gingerroot in large saucepan or Dutch oven. Bring to a boil. Reduce heat to medium. Add meatballs. Boil gently, uncovered, for 5 minutes. Reduce heat to medium-low.

Add noodles. Stir. Simmer, uncovered, for about 5 minutes until noodles are almost tender.

(continued on next page)

44   Soups, Salads & Dressings

Add bok choy. Stir. Simmer, uncovered, for about 2 minutes until tender-crisp.

Add green onion. Stir. Remove and discard gingerroot. Makes about 8 cups (2 L). Serves 6.

1 serving: 190 Calories; 5.6 g Total Fat (0.5 g Mono, 0.3 g Poly, 0.9 g Sat); 43 mg Cholesterol; 22 g Carbohydrate; 1 g Fibre; 13 g Protein; 440 mg Sodium

---

Chilled Beet Soup

A borscht by any other name is still a beet soup—but this chilled version delivers a whole new refreshing taste sensation.

Cans of whole baby beets (14 oz., 398 mL, each), with liquid	2	2
Prepared vegetable broth, chilled	1 1/2 cups	375 mL
Light sour cream	1/2 cup	125 mL
Chopped green onion	1/3 cup	75 mL
Chopped fresh dill (or 1 tbsp., 15 mL, dried)	1/4 cup	60 mL
Dill pickle juice	2 tbsp.	30 mL
Granulated sugar	1 tbsp.	15 mL
Pepper	1/4 tsp.	1 mL
Chopped dill pickle	2 tbsp.	30 mL

Put beets into large bowl. Mash until beets are crushed. Add next 7 ingredients. Stir well.

Stir in pickle. Makes about 6 cups (1.5 L). Serves 4.

1 serving: 122 Calories; 2.9 g Total Fat (trace Mono, trace Poly, 1.5 g Sat); 10 mg Cholesterol; 21 g Carbohydrate; 3 g Fibre; 4 g Protein; 896 mg Sodium

Variation: Heat soup in large saucepan on medium for about 8 minutes, stirring occasionally, until hot, but not boiling.

Chicken Curry Soup

Use up your leftover chicken in this irresistible coconut-flavoured
soup infused with a mild curry heat.

Canola oil	1 tsp.	5 mL
Chopped onion	1 cup	250 mL
Garlic cloves, minced	2	2
(or 1/2 tsp., 2 mL, powder)		
Low-sodium prepared chicken broth	4 cups	1 L
Brown sugar, packed	1 tbsp.	15 mL
Soy sauce	1 tbsp.	15 mL
Red curry paste	1/2 tsp.	2 mL
Frozen mixed Oriental vegetables,	2 cups	500 mL
larger pieces cut up		
Chopped cooked chicken breast	1 cup	250 mL
(see Tip, page 50)		
Light coconut milk	1/2 cup	125 mL
Lime juice	1 tbsp.	15 mL
Fish sauce (optional)	1 tsp.	5 mL

Heat canola oil in large saucepan or Dutch oven on medium. Add onion and garlic. Cook, uncovered, for about 5 minutes, stirring often, until onion starts to soften.

Add next 4 ingredients. Stir. Bring to a boil. Reduce heat to medium.

Add vegetables and chicken. Stir. Boil gently, uncovered, for about 5 minutes until vegetables are tender.

Add coconut milk. Stir. Remove from heat.

Add lime juice and fish sauce. Stir. Makes about 7 cups (1.75 L). Serves 6.

1 serving: 128 Calories; 3.8 g Total Fat (0.7 g Mono, 0.4 g Poly, 1.7 g Sat); 23 mg Cholesterol; 11 g Carbohydrate; 1 g Fibre; 11 g Protein; 450 mg Sodium

Pictured on page 53.

Spring Green Soup

Going green is a snap with this fresh, lemony dill soup packed with snow peas and asparagus.

Low-sodium prepared chicken broth	6 cups	1.5 L
Thinly sliced leek (white part only)	3/4 cup	175 mL
Vermicelli, broken up	4 oz.	113 g
Garlic clove, minced	1	1
(or 1/4 tsp., 1 mL, powder)		
Chopped fresh asparagus	1 cup	250 mL
Finely chopped low-fat deli ham	1 cup	250 mL
Snow peas, trimmed and halved	1 cup	250 mL
Chopped fresh dill (or 1 1/2 tsp, 7 mL, dried)	2 tbsp.	30 mL
Grated lemon zest	2 tsp.	10 mL

Measure broth into large saucepan. Bring to a boil.

Add next 3 ingredients. Stir. Boil, uncovered, for about 5 minutes, stirring occasionally, until pasta is almost tender.

Add next 3 ingredients. Stir. Cook, uncovered, for 2 to 4 minutes, stirring occasionally, until vegetables are tender-crisp.

Add dill and lemon zest. Stir. Makes about 7 1/2 cups (1.9 L). Serves 6.

1 serving: 174 Calories; 1.9 g Total Fat (trace Mono, 0.1 g Poly, 0.9 g Sat); 15 mg Cholesterol; 23 g Carbohydrate; 2 g Fibre; 15 g Protein; 641 mg Sodium

Pictured on page 53.

Paré Pointer

Is a fake diamond a shamrock?

Roasted Cauliflower Soup

Roasting the cauliflower adds an interesting dimension to this creamy-textured soup accented with a tangy red pepper drizzle.

Cauliflower florets	8 cups	2 L
Olive oil	2 tbsp.	30 mL
Dried thyme	1/4 tsp.	1 mL
Salt	1/2 tsp.	2 mL
Pepper	1/4 tsp.	1 mL
Prepared vegetable broth	3 cups	750 mL
Roasted red peppers	1/2 cup	125 mL
Prepared vegetable broth	1 tbsp.	15 mL
Dried basil	1/4 tsp.	1 mL

Preheat oven to 450°F (230°C). Put cauliflower into large bowl. Drizzle with olive oil. Sprinkle with next 3 ingredients. Toss until coated. Transfer to large ungreased baking sheet with sides. Spread evenly. Bake for about 15 minutes, stirring at halftime, until tender and starting to brown.

Meanwhile, measure first amount of broth into medium saucepan. Bring to a boil. Reduce heat to low. Cover to keep hot.

Put remaining 3 ingredients into blender or food processor. Process until smooth. Transfer to small cup. Rinse blender. Put cauliflower into blender. Add 2 cups (500 mL) hot broth. Process until smooth. Add to remaining hot broth. Stir. Makes about 5 1/2 cups (1.4 L) soup. Ladle into 4 soup bowls. Drizzle with red pepper mixture. Serves 4.

1 serving: 214 Calories; 8.0 g Total Fat (5.0 g Mono, 0.9 g Poly, 1.0 g Sat); trace Cholesterol; 31 g Carbohydrate; 13 g Fibre; 10 g Protein; 896 mg Sodium

Pictured on page 53.

Lemony Carrot Salad

Your daily ration of carrot sticks got you singing the blues? Change your tune with this delightful melody of carrots in a creamy lemony dressing.

Coarsely grated carrot	6 cups	1.5 L
Chopped fresh parsley, lightly packed	1/4 cup	60 mL
LEMON DRESSING		
Lemon juice	1/4 cup	60 mL
Liquid honey	1 tbsp.	15 mL
Small garlic clove, minced	1	1
(or 1/8 tsp., 0.5 mL, powder)		
Caraway seed	1/2 tsp.	2 mL
Salt	1/2 tsp.	2 mL
Cayenne pepper	1/8 tsp.	0.5 mL
Non-fat plain yogurt	3 tbsp.	50 mL
Olive oil	1 tbsp.	15 mL

Combine carrot and parsley in medium bowl.

Lemon Dressing: Combine first 6 ingredients in small bowl.

Whisk in yogurt and olive oil until combined. Makes about 2/3 cup (150 mL) dressing. Drizzle over carrot mixture. Toss until coated. Makes about 6 cups (1.5 L). Serves 6.

1 serving: 84 Calories; 2.6 g Total Fat (1.7 g Mono, 0.3 g Poly, 0.4 g Sat); trace Cholesterol; 15 g Carbohydrate; 3 g Fibre; 2 g Protein; 277 mg Sodium

Pictured on page 89.

Tropical Chicken Salad

The island flavours of coconut and pineapple combine to make a cool chicken salad that's sure to beat even the steamiest tropical heat.

Cut or torn romaine lettuce, lightly packed	4 cups	1 L
Chopped cooked chicken breast (see Tip, below)	2 1/2 cups	625 mL
Can of pineapple tidbits, drained and juice reserved	14 oz.	398 mL
Chopped unpeeled apple	1 cup	250 mL
Raisins	1/4 cup	60 mL
Shredded coconut	1/4 cup	60 mL
MINT DRESSING		
Chopped fresh mint (or 1 1/2 tsp., 7 mL, dried)	2 tbsp.	30 mL
Reserved pineapple juice	2 tbsp.	30 mL
Light mayonnaise	1 tbsp.	15 mL
Grated lime zest	1 tsp.	5 mL
Lime juice	1 tsp.	5 mL

Put first 6 ingredients into large bowl. Toss.

Mint Dressing: Combine all 5 ingredients in jar with tight-fitting lid. Shake well. Makes about 1/4 cup (60 mL) dressing. Drizzle over lettuce mixture. Toss. Makes about 9 cups (2.25 L). Serves 6.

1 serving: 194 Calories; 4.5 g Total Fat (1.2 g Mono, 0.8 g Poly, 1.8 g Sat); 50 mg Cholesterol; 20 g Carbohydrate; 3 g Fibre; 19 g Protein; 79 mg Sodium

 Don't have any leftover chicken? Start with 2 boneless, skinless chicken breast halves (4 – 6 oz., 113 – 170 g, each). Place in large frying pan with 1 cup (250 mL) water or chicken broth. Simmer, covered, for 12 to 14 minutes until no longer pink inside. Drain. Chop. Makes about 2 cups (500 mL) of cooked chicken.

Warm Couscous Salad

Is your dinner table always adorned with the same iceberg lettuce salad? Well, show family and friends your more daring self with this uniquely minty couscous salad speckled with cucumber and dates.

Water	1 3/4 cups	425 mL
Salt	1/4 tsp.	1 mL
Couscous	1 cup	250 mL
Chopped English cucumber (with peel)	2 cups	500 mL
Chopped pitted dates	1/2 cup	125 mL
Diced red pepper	1/2 cup	125 mL
Chopped green onion	1/4 cup	60 mL
Chopped fresh mint	2 tbsp.	30 mL
CHILI DRESSING		
Fat-free Italian dressing	1/3 cup	75 mL
Liquid honey	1 tbsp.	15 mL
Chili powder	1/2 tsp.	2 mL
Salt	1/4 tsp.	1 mL
Pepper	1/4 tsp.	1 mL

Combine water and salt in small saucepan. Bring to a boil. Add couscous. Stir. Remove from heat. Let stand, covered, for 5 minutes. Fluff with fork. Transfer to medium bowl.

Add next 5 ingredients. Toss.

Chili Dressing: Combine all 5 ingredients in jar with tight-fitting lid. Shake well. Makes about 1/3 cup (75 mL) dressing. Drizzle over couscous mixture. Toss. Makes about 6 cups (1.5 L). Serves 4.

1 serving: 279 Calories; 0.7 g Total Fat (0.1 g Mono, 0.2 g Poly, 0.2 g Sat); 1 mg Cholesterol; 62 g Carbohydrate; 4 g Fibre; 7 g Protein; 588 mg Sodium

Fast Bean Salad

This colourful mix of tender-crisp veggies and protein-packed beans makes a light and healthy lunch. For a nifty taste variation, substitute Roasted Red Pepper Dressing, page 56, for the Italian dressing.

Frozen cut green beans	1 cup	250 mL
Can of mixed beans, rinsed and drained	19 oz.	540 mL
Chopped celery	1/2 cup	125 mL
Chopped green onion	1/2 cup	125 mL
Chopped red pepper	1/2 cup	125 mL
Fat-free Italian dressing	1/4 cup	60 mL

Pour water into small saucepan until about 1 inch (2.5 cm) deep. Bring to a boil. Reduce heat to medium. Add green beans. Boil gently, covered, for about 2 minutes until tender-crisp. Immediately plunge into ice water in medium bowl. Let stand for about 5 minutes until cold. Drain.

Meanwhile, combine next 4 ingredients in large bowl. Drizzle with dressing. Add green beans. Toss until coated. Makes about 4 cups (1 L). Serves 4.

1 serving: 133 Calories; 0.8 g Total Fat (trace Mono, trace Poly, 0.1 g Sat); 1 mg Cholesterol; 26 g Carbohydrate; 7 g Fibre; 8 g Protein; 383 mg Sodium

Pictured on page 54.

1. Spring Green Soup, page 47
2. Roasted Cauliflower Soup, page 48
3. Chicken Curry Soup, page 46

Props courtesy of: Casa Bugatti

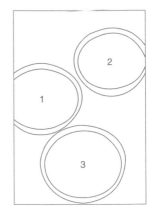

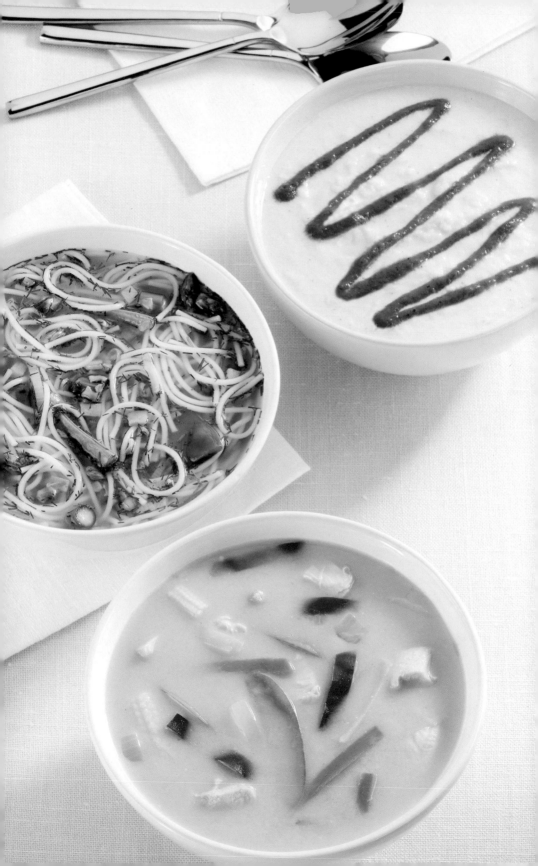

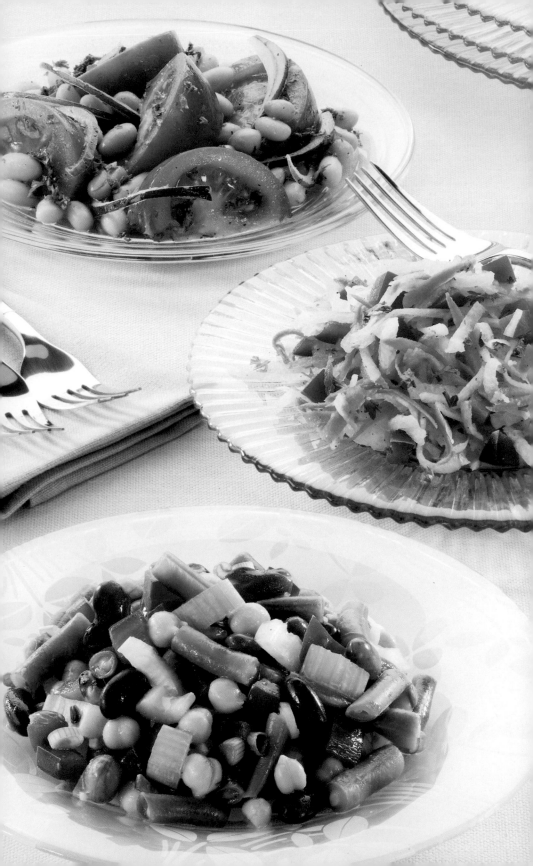

Jicama Coleslaw

Everyone's going to ask what the secret ingredient in your
crunchy coleslaw is. It's jicama (pronounced HEE-kah-mah).

Grated peeled jicama	3 cups	750 mL
Grated carrot	1 cup	250 mL
Diced red pepper	1/2 cup	125 mL
Chopped fresh parsley	2 tbsp.	30 mL
Finely diced red onion	2 tbsp.	30 mL
HONEY LIME DRESSING		
Lime juice	3 tbsp.	50 mL
Prepared vegetable broth	3 tbsp.	50 mL
Liquid honey	1 tbsp.	15 mL
Olive oil	1 tbsp.	15 mL
Pepper	1/4 tsp.	1 mL

Put first 5 ingredients into medium bowl. Toss.

Honey Lime Dressing: Combine all 5 ingredients in jar with tight-fitting lid. Shake well. Makes about 1/2 cup (125 mL) dressing. Drizzle over jicama mixture. Toss until coated. Makes about 4 cups (1 L). Serves 4.

1 serving: 107 Calories; 3.7 g Total Fat (2.5 g Mono, 0.4 g Poly, 0.5 g Sat); trace Cholesterol; 18 g Carbohydrate; 1 g Fibre; 1 g Protein; 62 mg Sodium

Pictured at left.

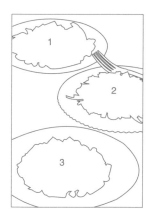

1. Tomato Salad, page 56
2. Jicama Coleslaw, above
3. Fast Bean Salad, page 52

Props courtesy of: Casa Bugatti

Tomato Salad

This lively tomato and kidney bean salad is at its absolute best when you use perfectly ripened tomatoes.

Can of white kidney beans, rinsed and drained	19 oz.	540 mL
Medium tomatoes, cut into 8 wedges each	4	4
Thinly sliced red (or sweet) onion	1/2 cup	125 mL
PARSLEY VINAIGRETTE		
Finely chopped fresh parsley, lightly packed	1/4 cup	60 mL
White vinegar	1/4 cup	60 mL
Olive (or canola) oil	2 tbsp.	30 mL
Granulated sugar	2 tsp.	10 mL
Ground cumin	1/4 tsp.	1 mL
Salt	1/8 tsp.	0.5 mL
Pepper	1/4 tsp.	1 mL

Put first 3 ingredients into large bowl.

Parsley Vinaigrette: Combine all 7 ingredients in jar with tight-fitting lid. Shake well. Makes about 1/2 cup (125 mL) vinaigrette. Drizzle over tomato mixture. Toss gently. Makes about 6 cups (1.5 L). Serves 6.

1 serving: 144 Calories; 5.6 g Total Fat (3.3 g Mono, 0.4 g Poly, 0.6 g Sat); 0 mg Cholesterol; 19 g Carbohydrate; 4 g Fibre; 5 g Protein; 82 mg Sodium

Pictured on page 54.

Roasted Red Pepper Dressing

We've jazzed up store-bought dressing and made it into something sensational!

Fat-free Italian dressing	1 cup	250 mL
Roasted red peppers	1/4 cup	60 mL
Grated light Parmesan cheese	2 tbsp.	30 mL

Put all 3 ingredients into blender or food processor. Process until smooth. Makes about 1 1/3 cups (325 mL).

2 tbsp. (30 mL): 29 Calories; 0.8 g Total Fat (0 g Mono, 0 g Poly, 0.1 g Sat); 3 mg Cholesterol; 4 g Carbohydrate; trace Fibre; 1 g Protein; 378 mg Sodium

Pictured on page 18.

Mango Dressing

*Dress your salad greens, veggie sticks and fresh fruit for success
with this very versatile, spicy mango dressing. Store in the fridge
in an airtight container for up to one week.*

Fat-free sour cream	1 cup	250 mL
Frozen mango pieces	1/2 cup	125 mL
Mango chutney	1/3 cup	75 mL
Apple cider vinegar	2 tbsp.	30 mL
Salt	1/2 tsp.	2 mL
Dried crushed chilies	1/4 tsp.	1 mL

Put all 6 ingredients into blender. Process until smooth. Makes about
1 1/3 cups (325 mL).

*2 tbsp. (30 mL): 81 Calories; 2.3 g Total Fat (trace Mono, trace Poly, trace Sat); 2 mg Cholesterol;
15 g Carbohydrate; trace Fibre; 1 g Protein; 364 mg Sodium*

Pictured on page 126.

Peanut Dressing

*Dressing, dip or all-time favourite new condiment. This Thai-inspired
topper goes with everything from greens to pork and chicken. Store
in the fridge in an airtight container for up to one week.*

Reduced-fat peanut butter	1/2 cup	125 mL
Water	1/2 cup	125 mL
Apple cider vinegar	3 tbsp.	50 mL
Brown sugar, packed	2 tbsp.	30 mL
Soy sauce	2 tbsp.	30 mL
Garlic cloves (or 1/2 tsp., 2 mL, powder)	2	2
Sesame oil (for flavour)	1/2 tsp.	2 mL

Put all 7 ingredients into blender. Process until smooth. Makes about
1 1/2 cups (375 mL).

*2 tbsp. (30 mL): 73 Calories; 4.0 g Total Fat (0.1 g Mono, 0.1 g Poly, 0.8 g Sat); 0 mg Cholesterol;
8 g Carbohydrate; 1 g Fibre; 3 g Protein; 207 mg Sodium*

SPICY PEANUT DRESSING: Add 1/2 tsp. (2 mL) chili paste (sambal oelek),
or 1/2 tsp. (2 mL) dried crushed chilies.

Meatloaf Patties

Make meatloaf more memorable by loading it with olives, sun-dried tomato pesto and roasted red peppers—all presented in handy single-serve portions.

White (or whole-wheat) bread slices, broken up	2	2
Skim milk	1/3 cup	75 mL
Extra-lean ground beef	1 lb.	454 g
Finely chopped onion	1/2 cup	125 mL
Finely chopped roasted red pepper	1/4 cup	60 mL
Ketchup	3 tbsp.	50 mL
Chopped black olives	2 tbsp.	30 mL
Sun-dried tomato pesto	2 tsp.	10 mL
Salt	1/2 tsp.	2 mL
Pepper	1/4 tsp.	1 mL

Put bread and milk into large bowl. Let stand until milk is absorbed.

Preheat broiler. Add remaining 8 ingredients to bread mixture. Mix well. Divide into 4 equal portions. Shape into 1/2 inch (12 mm) thick patties. Arrange on greased baking sheet with sides. Broil on top rack in oven for 6 to 8 minutes per side until fully cooked and internal temperature reaches 160°F (71°C). Serves 4.

1 serving: 254 Calories; 9.8 g Total Fat (3.5 g Mono, 0.5 g Poly, 3.3 g Sat); 61 mg Cholesterol; 14 g Carbohydrate; 1 g Fibre; 26 g Protein; 707 mg Sodium

Paré Pointer

Junk is something you've had for many years but throw out right before you need it.

Beef And Sweet Potato Ragout

Sweet potato adds an unexpected depth to this rich-tasting,
red wine-enhanced stew. Serve with egg noodles or rice.

Beef top sirloin steak, trimmed of fat	1 lb.	454 g
Seasoned salt	1/2 tsp.	2 mL
Pepper	1/4 tsp.	1 mL
Canola oil	1 tsp.	5 mL
Sliced fresh white mushrooms	2 cups	500 mL
Chopped onion	1/2 cup	125 mL
Garlic cloves, minced ,	2	2
(or 1/2 tsp., 2 mL powder)		
Dried rosemary, crushed	3/4 tsp.	4 mL
Cubed sweet potato	2 cups	500 mL
Prepared beef broth	1 cup	250 mL
Dry (or alcohol-free) red wine	1/2 cup	125 mL
Dijon mustard	2 tbsp.	30 mL
Worcestershire sauce	1 tsp.	5 mL
All-purpose flour	1 tbsp.	15 mL

Cut steak in half lengthwise. Cut halves crosswise into 1/4 inch (6 mm) thick slices, about 3 inches (7.5 cm) long. Sprinkle with seasoned salt and pepper. Heat canola oil in large frying pan on medium-high. Add beef. Cook for 2 to 3 minutes, stirring often, until desired doneness. Transfer to plate. Cover to keep warm.

Add next 4 ingredients to same frying pan. Heat and stir for 3 to 5 minutes until onion starts to soften.

Add next 5 ingredients. Stir. Bring to a boil. Reduce heat to medium. Cook, covered, for about 8 minutes until sweet potato is tender.

Stir 2 tbsp. (30 mL) cooking liquid into flour in small cup until smooth. Add to sweet potato mixture. Heat and stir until boiling and thickened. Add beef. Stir until heated through. Makes about 5 cups (1.25 L). Serves 4.

1 serving: 344 Calories; 9.6 g Total Fat (4.0 g Mono, 0.7 g Poly, 3.3 g Sat); 60 mg Cholesterol; 30 g Carbohydrate; 4 g Fibre; 28 g Protein; 644 mg Sodium

Pictured on page 89.

Orange Chili Beef

Take a dash of citrusy sweet paired with a dash of fiery chili heat, add some fresh tender-crisp veggies and you're on your way to a delicious stir-fry.

Orange juice	1 cup	250 mL
Cornstarch	1 tsp.	5 mL
Orange marmalade	2 tbsp.	30 mL
Finely grated gingerroot	1 tsp.	5 mL
(or 1/4 tsp., 1 mL, ground ginger)		
Grated orange zest	1 tsp.	5 mL
Garlic powder	1/2 tsp.	2 mL
Chili paste (sambal oelek)	1/4 tsp.	1 mL
Salt	1/2 tsp.	2 mL
Pepper	1/4 tsp.	1 mL
Canola oil	1 tsp.	5 mL
Beef top sirloin steak, trimmed of fat and cut into thin strips	3/4 lb.	340 g
Canola oil	1 tsp.	5 mL
Sliced onion	1 cup	250 mL
Sugar snap peas, trimmed	2 cups	500 mL
Sliced red pepper	1 cup	250 mL
Sliced yellow pepper	1 cup	250 mL

Stir orange juice into cornstarch in small bowl. Add next 7 ingredients. Mix well. Set aside.

Heat large frying pan or wok on medium-high until very hot. Add first amount of canola oil. Add beef. Stir-fry for about 2 minutes until no longer pink. Transfer to plate. Cover to keep warm.

Add second amount of canola oil to hot frying pan. Add onion. Stir-fry for 2 to 4 minutes until onion is tender-crisp.

Add remaining 3 ingredients. Stir cornstarch mixture. Add to vegetable mixture. Stir-fry for 2 to 3 minutes until vegetables are tender-crisp and sauce is thickened. Add beef. Stir until coated. Makes about 6 cups (1.5 L). Serves 4.

(continued on next page)

Beef & Pork

1 serving: 299 Calories; 8.7 g Total Fat (3.8 g Mono, 1.1 g Poly, 2.6 g Sat); 45 mg Cholesterol; 32 g Carbohydrate; 4 g Fibre; 23 g Protein; 360 mg Sodium

Pictured on page 89.

Chili-Rubbed Flank Steak

A quick and easy dry seasoning rub is all the
prep you need for a flavourful, juicy steak.

Chili powder	1 tsp.	5 mL
Ground cumin	1/4 tsp.	1 mL
Salt	1/2 tsp.	2 mL
Pepper	1/4 tsp.	1 mL
Ground cinnamon, just a pinch		
Flank steak, trimmed of fat	1 lb.	454 g
Cooking spray		

Preheat gas barbecue to medium (see Tip, page 64). Combine first 5 ingredients in small cup.

Rub spice mixture over steak. Spray with cooking spray. Cook on greased grill for 4 to 6 minutes per side until desired doneness. Transfer to cutting board. Cover with foil. Let stand for 5 minutes. Cut steak diagonally, across the grain, into 1/4 inch (6 mm) thick slices. Serves 4.

1 serving: 191 Calories; 8.8 g Total Fat (3.6 g Mono, 0.4 g Poly, 3.7 g Sat); 46 mg Cholesterol; trace Carbohydrate; trace Fibre; 26 g Protein; 354 mg Sodium

Pictured on page 89.

Peppery Balsamic Steaks

These steaks are beefed up with a sweet and spicy balsamic glaze—sure to please any meat lover!

Balsamic vinegar	3 tbsp.	50 mL
Liquid honey	3 tbsp.	50 mL
Dried crushed chilies	1/2 tsp.	2 mL
Beef top sirloin steak, cut into 4 equal portions	1 lb.	454 g
Montreal steak spice	1 tsp.	5 mL

Combine first 3 ingredients in small cup.

Score top of steak with sharp knife. Place steak in pie plate. Stir vinegar mixture. Pour over steak. Let stand for 5 minutes. Preheat broiler. Arrange steak on greased broiler pan. Brush with vinegar mixture.

Sprinkle 1/2 tsp. (2 mL) steak spice over top. Broil on top rack in oven for 5 minutes. Turn. Brush with vinegar mixture. Sprinkle remaining steak spice over top. Broil for another 2 to 4 minutes until desired doneness. Serves 4.

1 serving: 236 Calories; 8.1 g Total Fat (3.3 g Mono, 0.3 g Poly, 3.1 g Sat); 60 mg Cholesterol; 15 g Carbohydrate; trace Fibre; 24 g Protein; 174 mg Sodium

Pictured on page 107.

Paré Pointer

Don't trust pigs with secrets. They are the worst squealers around.

Beef & Pork

Speedy Beef Stew

A hearty, warming stew need not take hours to simmer.
This family-friendly favourite comes together in a flash.

Canola oil	2 tsp.	10 mL
Chopped onion	2 cups	500 mL
Extra-lean ground beef	1 lb.	454 g
Sliced carrot	1 cup	250 mL
Sliced celery	1 cup	250 mL
Chopped peeled potato	2 cups	500 mL
Water	1/4 cup	60 mL
All-purpose flour	3 tbsp.	50 mL
Prepared beef broth	2 cups	500 mL
Ketchup	1/4 cup	60 mL
Dried rosemary, crushed	1/2 tsp.	2 mL
Dried thyme	1/2 tsp.	2 mL
Salt	1/4 tsp.	1 mL
Pepper	1/2 tsp.	2 mL

Heat canola oil in large frying pan on medium-high. Add next 4 ingredients. Scramble-fry for 5 to 10 minutes until onion is softened. Drain.

Meanwhile, put potato and water into small microwave-safe bowl. Microwave, covered, on high (100%) for about 5 minutes until tender. Drain. Set aside.

Sprinkle flour over beef mixture. Heat and stir for 1 minute. Slowly add broth, stirring constantly, until smooth. Add remaining 5 ingredients. Heat and stir until boiling and thickened. Add potato. Stir. Simmer, covered, for 5 minutes to blend flavours. Makes about 6 cups (1.5 L). Serves 4.

1 serving: 375 Calories; 10.0 g Total Fat (4.5 g Mono, 1.0 g Poly, 3.5 g Sat); 60 mg Cholesterol; 44 g Carbohydrate; 5 g Fibre; 28 g Protein; 1293 mg Sodium

Sirloin Sizzle

*Add a little sizzle to your night with this tender steak basted
in a sweet and tangy homemade barbecue sauce.*

Beef top sirloin steak, trimmed of fat	1 lb.	454 g
Apple cider vinegar	3 tbsp.	50 mL
Ketchup	2 tbsp.	30 mL
Fancy (mild) molasses	1 tbsp.	15 mL
Steak sauce	1 tbsp.	15 mL
Dried oregano	1 tsp.	5 mL
Garlic clove, minced	1	1
(or 1/4 tsp., 1 mL, powder)		
Pepper	1/4 tsp.	1 mL
Ground cinnamon	1/8 tsp.	0.5 mL

Preheat gas barbecue to medium (see Tip, below). Place steak in pie plate.

Combine remaining 8 ingredients in small cup. Transfer 1 tbsp. (15 mL)
to small dish. Pour remaining vinegar mixture over steak. Turn to coat
both sides. Let stand for 10 minutes. Cook on greased grill for about
5 minutes per side until desired doneness. Transfer to cutting board.
Brush with reserved marinade. Cover with foil. Let stand for 5 minutes.
Cut into 4 equal portions. Serves 4.

*1 serving: 204 Calories; 8.1 g Total Fat (3.3 g Mono, 0.3 g Poly, 3.1 g Sat); 60 mg Cholesterol;
7 g Carbohydrate; trace Fibre; 25 g Protein; 196 mg Sodium*

 Too cold to barbecue? Use the broiler instead! Your food should cook
in about the same length of time—and remember to turn or baste as
directed. Set your oven rack so that the food is about 3 to 4 inches
(7.5 to 10 cm) away from the top element—for most ovens, this is
the top rack.

Raspberry Pork Tenderloin

Pork tenderloin is made all the sweeter when perfectly paired with an elegant lime-accented raspberry sauce. (Try the sauce on chicken, too!)

Pork tenderloin, trimmed of fat	1 lb.	454 g
Cooking spray		
Salt	1/2 tsp.	2 mL
Pepper	1/4 tsp.	1 mL
RASPBERRY SAUCE		
Canola oil	1/2 tsp.	2 mL
Chopped onion	1/2 cup	125 mL
Prepared chicken broth	1 cup	250 mL
Dry (or alcohol-free) white wine	1/4 cup	60 mL
Seedless raspberry jam	1/4 cup	60 mL
Water	2 tbsp.	30 mL
Cornstarch	2 tsp.	10 mL
Lime juice	1 tbsp.	15 mL

Preheat broiler. Place pork on greased wire rack set in baking sheet with sides. Spray with cooking spray. Sprinkle with salt and pepper. Broil on centre rack in oven for about 5 minutes until starting to brown. Turn on oven to 450°F (230°C). Bake for about 20 minutes until internal temperature reaches 160°F (71°C). Transfer to cutting board. Cover with foil.

Raspberry Sauce: Meanwhile, heat canola oil in small saucepan on medium. Add onion. Cook for about 5 minutes, stirring occasionally, until onion starts to soften.

Add next 3 ingredients. Stir. Bring to a boil. Reduce heat to medium. Boil gently, uncovered, for about 5 minutes until smooth.

Stir water into cornstarch in small cup. Add to jam mixture. Heat and stir until boiling and thickened. Remove from heat.

Add lime juice. Stir. Makes about 1 cup (250 mL) sauce. Cut pork into 1/2 inch (12 mm) thick slices. Serve with Raspberry Sauce. Serves 4.

1 serving: 231 Calories; 5.7 g Total Fat (2.6 g Mono, 0.8 g Poly, 1.8 g Sat); 71 mg Cholesterol; 17 g Carbohydrate; trace Fibre; 24 g Protein; 723 mg Sodium

Pork Strip Goulash

We used a slick trick to drastically cut the calories and fat in this creamy classic—instead of regular cooking oil, we've used low-fat Italian dressing (with the added benefit of built-in spices!).

Boneless centre-cut pork chops, trimmed of fat	1 lb.	454 g
Low-fat Italian dressing	2 tbsp.	30 mL
Seasoned salt	1 tsp.	5 mL
Low-fat Italian dressing	1 tbsp.	15 mL
Chopped onion	1 cup	250 mL
Garlic clove, minced (or 1/4 tsp., 1 mL, powder)	1	1
Paprika	1 tsp.	5 mL
Prepared chicken broth	1 cup	250 mL
Skim evaporated milk	1 cup	250 mL
All-purpose flour	1 1/2 tbsp.	25 mL
Roasted red pepper, chopped	1/2 cup	125 mL
Fat-free sour cream	1/2 cup	125 mL

Cut pork crosswise into 1/4 inch (6 mm) thick slices. Cut slices lengthwise into thin strips. Put into medium bowl. Drizzle with first amount of dressing. Sprinkle with seasoned salt. Toss until coated. Heat large frying pan on medium-high until very hot. Add pork mixture. Stir-fry for about 5 minutes until pork is no longer pink. Transfer to plate. Cover to keep warm. Reduce heat to medium.

Add next 3 ingredients to same frying pan. Cook for 3 to 5 minutes, stirring often, until onion starts to soften. Sprinkle with paprika. Heat and stir for 1 minute.

Add broth. Stir. Bring to a boil.

Whisk evaporated milk into flour in small bowl until smooth. Slowly add to broth mixture, stirring constantly, until boiling and thickened.

Add red pepper and pork. Heat and stir for 1 to 2 minutes until heated through.

(continued on next page)

Beef & Pork

Stir in sour cream. Makes about 4 1/2 cups (1.1 L). Serves 4.

1 serving: 300 Calories; 10.0 g Total Fat (2.9 g Mono, 0.6 g Poly, 3.9 g Sat); 73 mg Cholesterol; 19 g Carbohydrate; 2 g Fibre; 31 g Protein; 1063 mg Sodium

Not-So-Portly Pork

Is your year's bounty of rhubarb really starting to pile up? Take advantage of pork's ability to go well with all things sweet and tart, and use it in this tangy taste temptation.

Canola oil	1 tsp.	5 mL
Boneless pork loin chops, trimmed of fat (about 1 lb., 454 g)	4	4
Port wine	1/4 cup	60 mL
Sliced fresh rhubarb	1 1/2 cups	375 mL
Granulated sugar	3 tbsp.	50 mL
Finely grated gingerroot (or 1/4 tsp., 1 mL, ground ginger)	1 tsp.	5 mL

Heat canola oil in large frying pan on medium-high. Add pork. Cook for about 2 minutes per side until browned. Reduce heat to medium-low.

Add wine. Heat and stir for 15 seconds, scraping any brown bits from bottom of pan.

Combine remaining 3 ingredients in small bowl. Add to pork mixture. Stir. Cook, covered, for 8 to 10 minutes, turning pork at halftime, until desired doneness. Transfer pork to serving dish. Spoon rhubarb mixture over top. Serves 4.

1 serving: 238 Calories; 7.6 g Total Fat (3.6 g Mono, 0.8 g Poly, 2.4 g Sat); 65 mg Cholesterol; 13 g Carbohydrate; 1 g Fibre; 24 g Protein; 51 mg Sodium

Mango Fennel Pork

The unexpected duo of mango and fennel combine creatively for an enticingly delicious sauce for tender pork. Any dinner guest would be duly impressed!

Crushed fennel seed	1 tsp.	5 mL
Pepper	1/2 tsp.	2 mL
Pork tenderloin, trimmed of fat and cut into 1/2 inch (12 mm) thick slices	1 lb.	454 g
Canola oil	2 tsp.	10 mL
Canola oil	1 tsp.	5 mL
Sliced onion	1 cup	250 mL
Finely grated gingerroot	2 tsp.	10 mL
Garlic cloves, minced (or 1/2 tsp., 2 mL, powder)	2	2
All-purpose flour	1 tbsp.	15 mL
Mango nectar	1/2 cup	125 mL
Prepared chicken broth	1/2 cup	125 mL
Salt	1/2 tsp.	2 mL
Chopped frozen mango pieces, thawed	2 cups	500 mL
Chopped fresh parsley	2 tbsp.	30 mL

Sprinkle fennel seed and pepper over pork. Heat first amount of canola oil in large frying pan on medium-high. Add pork. Cook for 2 to 3 minutes per side until browned. Transfer to plate. Cover to keep warm. Reduce heat to medium.

Add second amount of canola oil to same frying pan. Add next 3 ingredients. Cook for 3 to 5 minutes, stirring often, until onion is softened.

Sprinkle with flour. Heat and stir for 1 minute.

Add next 3 ingredients. Heat and stir until boiling and slightly thickened.

Add mango and pork. Cook, covered, for about 3 minutes until pork is no longer pink inside. Transfer pork to serving dish. Pour mango mixture over top.

Sprinkle with parsley. Serves 4.

1 serving: 276 Calories; 8.7 g Total Fat (4.4 g Mono, 1.6 g Poly, 2.0 g Sat); 71 mg Cholesterol; 24 g Carbohydrate; 2 g Fibre; 25 g Protein; 542 mg Sodium

Pictured on page 71 and back cover.

Glazed Pork Chops

Pork, plum and a little bit of spice are the
perfect combo in this easy Asian-style dish.

Canola oil	1 tsp.	5 mL
Boneless centre-cut pork chops, trimmed of fat (about 1 lb., 454 g)	4	4
Salt	1/4 tsp.	1 mL
Pepper	1/4 tsp.	1 mL
Chopped green pepper	1 cup	250 mL
Chopped onion	1 cup	250 mL
Finely grated gingerroot (or 1/2 tsp., 2 mL, ground ginger)	2 tsp.	10 mL
Plum sauce	2/3 cup	150 mL
Orange juice	2 tbsp.	30 mL
Grated orange zest	1 tsp.	5 mL
Dried crushed chilies	1/2 tsp.	2 mL

Heat canola oil in large frying pan on medium-high. Sprinkle pork with salt and pepper. Add to frying pan. Cook for 2 to 3 minutes per side until no longer pink inside. Transfer to large plate. Cover to keep warm. Reduce heat to medium.

Add next 3 ingredients to same frying pan. Cook for 3 to 5 minutes, stirring often, until green pepper and onion are tender-crisp.

Add remaining 4 ingredients and pork. Cook for 2 to 4 minutes, turning pork to coat both sides, until heated through. Serves 4.

1 serving: 301 Calories; 8.6 g Total Fat (3.9 g Mono, 1.4 g Poly, 2.5 g Sat); 62 mg Cholesterol; 28 g Carbohydrate; 2 g Fibre; 26 g Protein; 468 mg Sodium

Pictured on page 71 and on back cover.

Pork Bean Stew

Kids and adults alike will be satisfied with our refined version of pork 'n' beans. Serve with a crusty loaf of bread or thick toast slices.

Canola oil	1 tsp.	5 mL
Chopped onion	2 cups	500 mL
Pork tenderloin, trimmed of fat and diced	1 lb.	454 g
Diced red pepper	1 cup	250 mL
Paprika	1 tbsp.	15 mL
Can of tomato sauce	25 oz.	680 mL
Can of mixed beans, rinsed and drained	19 oz.	540 mL
Granulated sugar	2 tbsp.	30 mL
Garlic and herb no-salt seasoning	1 tbsp.	15 mL

Heat canola oil in large frying pan on medium-high. Add next 4 ingredients. Cook for 5 to 10 minutes, stirring often, until onion starts to soften.

Add remaining 4 ingredients. Stir. Bring to a boil. Reduce heat to medium-low. Simmer, partially covered, for about 5 minutes, stirring occasionally, until slightly thickened and pork reaches desired doneness. Makes about 8 cups (2 L). Serves 6.

1 serving: 255 Calories; 4.8 g Total Fat (1.9 g Mono, 0.8 g Poly, 1.2 g Sat); 48 mg Cholesterol; 33 g Carbohydrate; 7 g Fibre; 23 g Protein; 859 mg Sodium

Pictured at right and on back cover.

1. Mango Fennel Pork, page 68
2. Pork Bean Stew, above
3. Glazed Pork Chops, page 69

Props courtesy of: Danesco Inc.
The Bay
Winners Stores

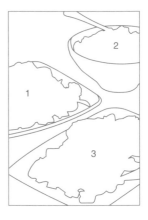

Beef & Pork

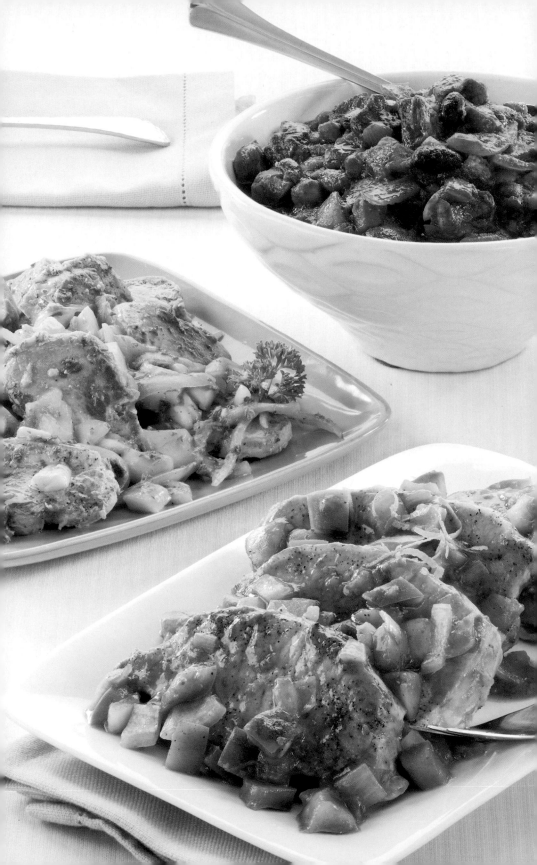

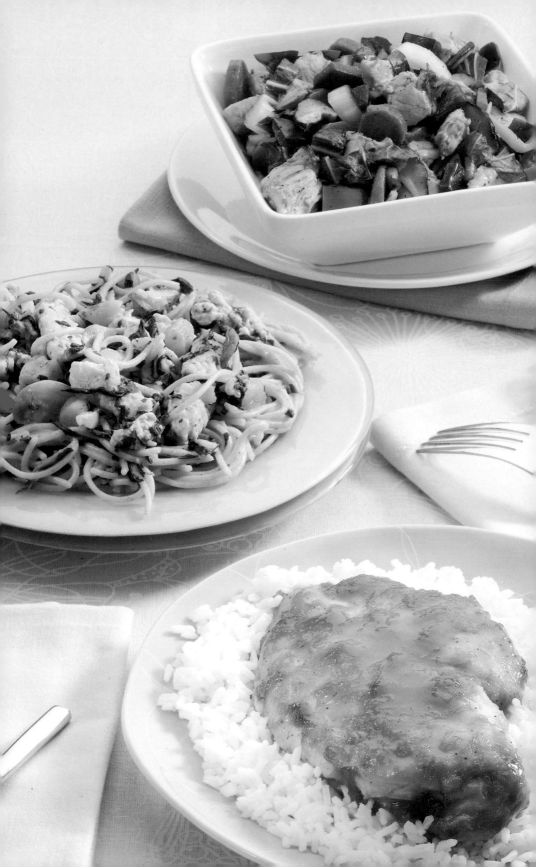

Chicken Chili

With smoky chipotle peppers, this treat will hold its own at any chili cook-off.

Canola oil	1 tsp.	5 mL
Lean ground chicken breast	1 lb.	454 g
Chopped celery	1 cup	250 mL
Chopped green pepper	1 cup	250 mL
Chopped onion	1 cup	250 mL
Chili powder	1 tsp.	5 mL
Chopped chipotle pepper in adobo sauce (see Tip, page 26)	1 tsp.	5 mL
Garlic powder	1/4 tsp.	1 mL
Ground cumin	1/4 tsp.	1 mL
Salt	1/4 tsp.	1 mL
Pepper	1/4 tsp.	1 mL
Can of tomato sauce	25 oz.	680 mL
Can of diced tomatoes, drained	14 oz.	398 mL
Can of red kidney beans, rinsed and drained	14 oz.	398 mL

Heat canola oil in large saucepan or Dutch oven on medium-high. Add next 10 ingredients. Scramble-fry for about 5 minutes until chicken is no longer pink.

Add remaining 3 ingredients. Bring to a boil. Reduce heat to medium-low. Simmer, uncovered, for 2 to 3 minutes until heated through. Makes about 8 cups (2 L). Serves 6.

1 serving: 391 Calories; 4.1 g Total Fat (1.4 g Mono, 1.3 g Poly, 0.9 g Sat); 44 mg Cholesterol; 56 g Carbohydrate; 13 g Fibre; 34 g Protein; 1039 mg Sodium

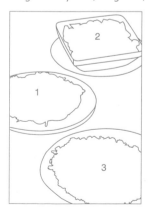

1. Apricot Turkey Pasta, page 84
2. Chicken Hotpot, page 74
3. Lemon Ginger Chicken, page 75

Props courtesy of: Pier 1 Imports

Chicken Hotpot

Tender-crisp carrots, bamboo shoots and bok choy make
an outstanding appearance in this mildly hot and tangy hotpot.

Canola oil	2 tsp.	10 mL
Boneless, skinless chicken breast halves, chopped	3/4 lb.	340 g
Sliced carrot	1 cup	250 mL
Sliced fresh shiitake mushrooms	1 cup	250 mL
Can of shoestring-style sliced bamboo shoots, drained	8 oz.	227 mL
Prepared chicken broth	1/4 cup	60 mL
Rice vinegar	1/4 cup	60 mL
Soy sauce	2 tbsp.	30 mL
Granulated sugar	2 tsp.	10 mL
Finely grated gingerroot	1 tsp.	5 mL
Sesame oil (for flavour)	1 tsp.	5 mL
Pepper	1/2 tsp.	2 mL
Sliced bok choy	2 cups	500 mL
Chopped red pepper	1 cup	250 mL
Water	2 tbsp.	30 mL
Cornstarch	1 tbsp.	15 mL

Heat canola oil in large saucepan on medium-high. Add chicken. Cook, uncovered, for 2 to 4 minutes, stirring occasionally, until no longer pink.

Add next 10 ingredients. Stir. Bring to a boil. Reduce heat to medium. Boil gently, partially covered, for 2 to 4 minutes until carrot is almost tender-crisp.

Add bok choy and red pepper. Stir. Cook, covered, for 2 to 4 minutes until vegetables are tender-crisp.

Stir water into cornstarch in small cup. Add to chicken mixture. Heat and stir until boiling and thickened. Makes about 6 cups (1.5 L). Serves 4.

1 serving: 189 Calories; 5.3 g Total Fat (2.1 g Mono, 1.7 g Poly, 0.8 g Sat); 49 mg Cholesterol; 13 g Carbohydrate; 3 g Fibre; 23 g Protein; 543 mg Sodium

Pictured on page 72.

Lemon Ginger Chicken

Different yet familiar, soothing yet refreshing—you'll wish you'd discovered this fine flavour combination sooner. Serve with rice or noodles.

Boneless, skinless chicken breast halves (4 – 6 oz., 113 – 170 g, each)	4	4
All-purpose flour	1/4 cup	60 mL
Salt	1/4 tsp.	1 mL
Pepper	1/4 tsp.	1 mL
Olive (or canola) oil	2 tsp.	10 mL
Prepared chicken broth	1/2 cup	125 mL
Lemon juice	1/4 cup	60 mL
Brown sugar, packed	2 tbsp.	30 mL
Soy sauce	1 tbsp.	15 mL
Finely grated gingerroot	1 tsp.	5 mL
Grated lemon zest	1 tsp.	5 mL
Dry mustard	1/4 tsp.	1 mL
Prepared chicken broth	1/4 cup	60 mL
Cornstarch	1 1/2 tsp.	7 mL

Place chicken between 2 sheets of plastic wrap. Pound with mallet or rolling pin to 1/4 inch (6 mm) thickness. Combine next 3 ingredients on large plate. Press both sides of chicken into flour mixture until coated. Discard any remaining flour mixture.

Heat olive oil in large frying pan on medium-high. Add chicken. Cook for 2 to 4 minutes per side until no longer pink inside. Transfer to plate. Cover to keep warm. Reduce heat to medium.

Add next 7 ingredients to same frying pan. Heat and stir, scraping any brown bits from bottom of pan, until boiling.

Stir second amount of broth into cornstarch in small cup. Add to lemon juice mixture. Heat and stir until boiling and thickened. Reduce heat to medium-low. Add chicken. Turn to coat both sides. Cook for 1 to 2 minutes until heated through. Serves 4.

1 serving: 232 Calories; 4.8 g Total Fat (2.3 g Mono, 0.8 g Poly, 1.0 g Sat); 82 mg Cholesterol; 12 g Carbohydrate; trace Fibre; 33 g Protein; 632 mg Sodium

Pictured on page 72.

Chicken Porcini Parcels

The rich flavour of porcini mushrooms ensure
these petite parcels pack a wallop of flavour.

Package of dried porcini mushrooms	1/2 oz.	14 g
Boiling water	1 cup	250 mL
Dry sherry	3 tbsp.	50 mL
Dried rosemary, crushed	1/2 tsp.	2 mL
Light herb and garlic cream cheese	1/4 cup	60 mL
Chicken breast cutlets (about 1 lb., 454 g)	4	4
Salt, sprinkle		
Pepper, sprinkle		
Chopped fresh parsley	2 tbsp.	30 mL

Preheat oven to 450°F (230°C). Put mushrooms into small heatproof bowl. Add boiling water. Stir. Let stand, covered, for about 5 minutes until softened. Drain. Chop coarsely.

Heat small frying pan on medium. Add sherry, rosemary and mushrooms. Cook for 2 to 4 minutes until liquid is almost evaporated.

Add cream cheese. Stir until melted.

Cut 4 sheets of heavy-duty (or double layer of regular) foil, about 14 inches long each. Spray one side of each sheet with cooking spray. Place 1 piece of chicken in centre of each sheet. Sprinkle with salt and pepper. Spoon mushroom mixture over chicken. Fold edges of foil together over chicken to enclose. Fold ends to seal completely. Place, seam-side up, on baking sheet. Bake for about 10 minutes until chicken is no longer pink inside. Remove chicken from foil.

Sprinkle with parsley. Serves 4.

1 serving: 178 Calories; 4.3 g Total Fat (0.5 g Mono, 0.5 g Poly, 2.0 g Sat); 76 mg Cholesterol; 4 g Carbohydrate; 1 g Fibre; 28 g Protein; 146 mg Sodium

Thai Coconut Chicken

Thai this on for size! With the mingling of such delightful
flavours as peanut, coconut, chili and lime, this delectable
dinner is a pleasant alternative to the norm.

Prepared chicken broth	1 1/4 cups	300 mL
Lime juice	3 tbsp.	50 mL
Soy sauce	2 tbsp.	30 mL
Finely grated gingerroot	1 tbsp.	15 mL
Grated lime zest (see Tip, page 30)	1 tbsp.	15 mL
Garlic cloves, minced	2	2
(or 1/2 tsp., 2 mL, powder)		
Pepper	1/4 tsp.	1 mL
Boneless, skinless chicken breast halves	4	4
(4 – 6 oz., 113 – 170 g, each)		
Brown sugar, packed	1/4 cup	60 mL
Reduced-fat peanut butter	2 tbsp.	30 mL
Sweet chili sauce	1 tbsp.	15 mL
Light coconut milk	1/2 cup	125 mL
Cornstarch	2 tsp.	10 mL

Combine first 7 ingredients in medium frying pan. Bring to a boil. Reduce heat to medium.

Add chicken. Cook, covered, for 12 to 15 minutes, turning at halftime, until chicken is no longer pink inside. Transfer chicken to plate. Cover to keep warm.

Whisk next 3 ingredients into broth mixture until smooth. Bring to a boil.

Stir coconut milk into cornstarch in small cup. Slowly add to broth mixture, stirring constantly with whisk, until boiling and slightly thickened. Serve with chicken. Serves 4.

1 serving: 304 Calories; 7.6 g Total Fat (0.7 g Mono, 0.7 g Poly, 2.7 g Sat); 82 mg Cholesterol;
22 g Carbohydrate; 1 g Fibre; 35 g Protein; 1012 mg Sodium

Orange Cumin Chicken

Baking in foil intensifies this chicken's orange and cumin flavours.

Frozen concentrated orange juice, thawed	1/4 cup	60 mL
Brown sugar, packed	1 tbsp.	15 mL
Ground cumin	1 tsp.	5 mL
Garlic powder	1/2 tsp.	2 mL
Ground cinnamon	1/2 tsp.	2 mL
Ground ginger	1/2 tsp.	2 mL
Sesame oil (for flavour)	1/2 tsp.	2 mL
Salt	1/2 tsp.	2 mL
Pepper	1/2 tsp.	2 mL
Boneless, skinless chicken breast halves (4 – 6 oz., 113 – 170 g, each)	4	4

Preheat oven to 450°F (230°C). Combine first 9 ingredients in small bowl.

Cut 4 sheets of heavy-duty (or double layer of regular) foil, about 14 inches long each. Place 1 chicken breast in centre of each sheet. Spoon orange juice mixture over top. Fold edges of foil together over chicken to enclose. Fold ends to seal completely. Place seam-side up, on baking sheet. Bake for 18 to 20 minutes until chicken is fully cooked and internal temperature reaches 170°F (77°C). Serves 4.

1 serving: 179 Calories; 2.6 g Total Fat (0.7 g Mono, 0.7 g Poly, 0.6 g Sat); 66 mg Cholesterol; 11 g Carbohydrate; trace Fibre; 26 g Protein; 358 mg Sodium

Ginger Mango Chicken

Heat up your evening with these sweet and gingery chicken cutlets.

Canola oil	2 tsp.	10 mL
Chicken breast cutlets (about 1 lb., 454 g)	4	4
Salt	1/4 tsp.	1 mL
Pepper	1/4 tsp.	1 mL
Mango chutney, larger pieces chopped	1/2 cup	125 mL
Orange juice	1/4 cup	60 mL
Finely grated gingerroot	1 1/2 tsp.	7 mL
Ground allspice	1/4 tsp.	1 mL

(continued on next page)

Heat canola oil in large frying pan on medium-high. Add chicken. Sprinkle with salt and pepper. Cook for about 2 minutes per side until browned.

Meanwhile, combine remaining 4 ingredients in small bowl. Pour over chicken. Reduce heat to low. Cook, covered, for about 5 minutes until chicken is no longer pink inside. Serves 4.

1 serving: 237 Calories; 7.3 g Total Fat (1.8 g Mono, 1.1 g Poly, 0.7 g Sat); 66 mg Cholesterol; 17 g Carbohydrate; 1 g Fibre; 26 g Protein; 523 mg Sodium

Honey Dijon Lemon Chicken

With its delicate and mildly sweet sauce, this elegant chicken dish is perfect to serve when you're set on impressing even the most refined diners.

Canola oil	1 tsp.	5 mL
Boneless, skinless chicken breast halves (4 – 6 oz., 113 – 170 g, each)	4	4
Prepared chicken broth	1 1/2 cups	375 mL
Liquid honey	1/4 cup	60 mL
Dijon mustard	2 tbsp.	30 mL
Lemon juice	1 tbsp.	15 mL
Grated lemon zest	1/2 tsp.	2 mL
Pepper	1/4 tsp.	1 mL
Prepared chicken broth	2 tbsp.	30 mL
Cornstarch	2 tsp.	10 mL
Half-and-half cream	1/2 cup	125 mL

Heat canola oil in medium frying pan on medium-high. Add chicken. Cook for 2 to 3 minutes per side until browned.

Add next 6 ingredients. Bring to a boil on medium. Cook, covered, for 12 to 15 minutes until no longer pink inside. Transfer chicken to plate. Cover to keep warm.

Stir second amount of broth into cornstarch in small cup. Add to honey mixture. Heat and stir until boiling and thickened. Stir in cream. Cook for 1 minute. Serve with chicken. Serves 4.

1 serving: 261 Calories; 7.1 g Total Fat (2.3 g Mono, 1.0 g Poly, 2.9 g Sat); 78 mg Cholesterol; 21 g Carbohydrate; trace Fibre; 27 g Protein; 776 mg Sodium

Pictured on page 18.

Red Pepper Chicken

The unpredicted pairing of tangy lemon with pepper sauce
yields delicious results in this moist chicken dish.

Large lemon	1	1
Water	1 1/2 cups	375 mL
Gingerroot slices (1/4 inch, 6 mm, thick)	4	4
Garlic clove, sliced	1	1
Boneless, skinless chicken breast halves (4 – 6 oz., 113 – 170 g, each)	4	4
Diced red pepper	1 cup	250 mL
Garlic clove, minced (or 1/4 tsp., 1 mL, powder)	1	1
Granulated sugar	1/3 cup	75 mL
Soy sauce	3 tbsp.	50 mL
Cornstarch	2 tbsp.	30 mL
Hot pepper sauce	1/4 tsp.	1 mL
Chopped fresh cilantro or parsley	2 tbsp.	30 mL

Cut lemon in half. Squeeze juice into small cup. Set aside. Put squeezed lemon halves into large frying pan.

Add next 3 ingredients. Bring to a boil. Reduce heat to medium. Add chicken. Cook, covered, for 12 to 15 minutes, turning at halftime, until chicken is no longer pink inside. Transfer chicken to plate. Cover to keep warm. Strain liquid. Discard solids. Return liquid to same frying pan. Bring to a boil.

Add red pepper and garlic. Cook for about 1 minute until fragrant.

Measure 1/3 cup (75 mL) lemon juice into small bowl. Add next 4 ingredients. Stir until smooth. Slowly add to frying pan, stirring constantly, until boiling and thickened.

Add cilantro and chicken. Cook and stir for about 1 minute until heated through. Serves 4.

1 serving: 264 Calories; 2.4 g Total Fat (0.6 g Mono, 0.6 g Poly, 0.6 g Sat); 82 mg Cholesterol; 26 g Carbohydrate; 1 g Fibre; 34 g Protein; 681 mg Sodium

Saucy Sausage Supper

This bold and spicy spaghetti dish is made all the more saucy with the cheeky addition of fennel—and using a box of pasta makes it all the more convenient.

Water	13 cups	3.25 L
Salt	1 1/2 tsp.	7 mL
Whole-wheat spaghetti	13 oz.	370 g
Canola oil	1 tsp.	5 mL
Turkey (or chicken) sausage, casing removed	13 oz.	370 g
Chopped onion	1/2 cup	125 mL
Fennel seed	1 tsp.	5 mL
Sliced fresh white mushrooms	2 cups	500 mL
Small zucchini (with peel), halved lengthwise and thinly sliced	2	2
Can of diced tomatoes (with juice)	28 oz.	796 mL
Tomato paste (see Tip, page 83)	1 tbsp.	15 mL
Grated light Parmesan cheese	2 tbsp.	30 mL

Combine water and salt in Dutch oven or large pot. Bring to a boil. Add spaghetti. Boil, uncovered, for 10 to 12 minutes, stirring occasionally, until tender but firm. Drain. Return to same pot. Cover to keep warm.

Meanwhile, heat canola oil in large frying pan on medium-high. Add next 3 ingredients. Scramble-fry for about 5 minutes until sausage is no longer pink and onion is softened.

Add mushrooms and zucchini. Cook for about 5 minutes, stirring occasionally, until vegetables start to soften. Drain.

Add tomatoes with juice and tomato paste. Stir. Cook, partially covered, for 8 minutes to blend flavours. Add to pasta. Stir until coated.

Sprinkle with cheese. Makes about 10 cups (2.5 L). Serves 6.

1 serving: 375 Calories; 7.7 g Total Fat (2.0 g Mono, 1.9 g Poly, 1.3 g Sat); 48 mg Cholesterol; 58 g Carbohydrate; 6 g Fibre; 24 g Protein; 761 mg Sodium

Cajun Chicken

This corn and red pepper-spiked chicken dish offers just the right amount of heat to pleasantly tantalize the taste buds. Serve with cornbread.

Boneless, skinless chicken breast halves, cut into 1 inch (2.5 cm) cubes	1 lb.	454 g
Cajun seasoning	1 tbsp.	15 mL
Garlic powder	1/2 tsp.	2 mL
Salt	1/2 tsp.	2 mL
Canola oil	1 tsp.	5 mL
Chopped onion	1 cup	250 mL
Chopped red pepper	1 cup	250 mL
Frozen kernel corn	1 cup	250 mL
Cajun seasoning	1/2 tsp.	2 mL
Salt	1/4 tsp.	1 mL
Pepper	1/8 tsp.	0.5 mL
Chopped tomato	1 cup	250 mL

Put chicken into medium bowl. Sprinkle with next 3 ingredients. Toss until coated.

Heat canola oil in medium frying pan on medium-high. Add onion and chicken. Cook for 5 to 8 minutes, stirring occasionally, until chicken is browned.

Add next 5 ingredients. Stir. Cook for about 2 minutes, stirring occasionally, until red pepper is tender-crisp.

Add tomato. Stir. Cook for about 1 minute until tomato starts to soften. Makes about 5 cups (1.25 L). Serves 4.

1 serving: 203 Calories; 3.4 g Total Fat (1.1 g Mono, 0.9 g Poly, 0.6 g Sat); 66 mg Cholesterol; 15 g Carbohydrate; 3 g Fibre; 28 g Protein; 980 mg Sodium

Turkey Burgers

Choose turkey for a hearty, yet low-fat alternative to regular beef burgers.
Dress up these beauties with fat-free condiments like ketchup and salsa.

Fine dry bread crumbs	1/4 cup	60 mL
Dijon mustard	1 tbsp.	15 mL
Prepared horseradish	1 tbsp.	15 mL
Paprika	1 tsp.	5 mL
Pepper	1/4 tsp.	1 mL
Salt	1/8 tsp.	0.5 mL
Extra-lean ground turkey thigh	1 lb.	454 g
Butter lettuce leaves	4	4
Tomato slices	4	4
Onion buns, split	4	4

Preheat broiler. Combine first 6 ingredients in medium bowl.

Add turkey. Mix well. Divide into 4 equal portions. Shape into 1/2 inch (12 mm) thick patties. Arrange on greased broiler pan. Broil on top rack in oven for 4 to 5 minutes per side until fully cooked and internal temperature reaches 175°F (80°C).

Serve patties, topped with lettuce and tomato, in buns. Serves 4.

1 serving: 306 Calories; 4.5 g Total Fat (0.2 g Mono, 0.2 g Poly, 1.1 g Sat); 45 mg Cholesterol; 32 g Carbohydrate; 2 g Fibre; 35 g Protein; 509 mg Sodium

 tip If a recipe calls for less than an entire can of tomato paste, freeze the unopened can for 30 minutes. Open both ends and push the contents through one end. Slice off only what you need. Freeze the remaining paste in a resealable freezer bag or plastic wrap for future use.

Apricot Turkey Pasta

This light yet creamy dinner delight has the added benefits of sweet apricot and tender turkey. Pasta lovers will leave the table well satisfied.

Water	12 cups	3 L
Salt	1 1/2 tsp.	7 mL
Whole-wheat spaghetti	8 oz.	225 g
Canola oil	2 tsp.	10 mL
Turkey breast cutlets, cut into thin strips (see Note)	1 lb.	454 g
Canola oil	2 tsp.	10 mL
Sliced fresh white mushrooms	1 cup	250 mL
Chopped onion	1/2 cup	125 mL
All-purpose flour	2 tbsp.	30 mL
Skim milk	2 cups	500 mL
Box of frozen chopped spinach, thawed and squeezed dry	10 oz.	300 g
Chopped dried apricot	1/2 cup	125 mL
Ground nutmeg	1/4 tsp.	1 mL
Salt	1/2 tsp.	2 mL
Pepper	1/4 tsp.	1 mL
Grated lemon zest	2 tsp.	10 mL

Combine water and salt in Dutch oven. Bring to a boil. Add spaghetti. Boil, uncovered, for 10 to 12 minutes, stirring occasionally, until tender but firm. Drain. Return to same pot. Cover to keep warm.

Meanwhile, heat first amount of canola oil in large frying pan on medium-high. Add turkey. Cook for 3 to 5 minutes, stirring occasionally, until browned. Transfer to plate. Cover to keep warm. Reduce heat to medium.

Add second amount of canola oil to same frying pan. Add mushrooms and onion. Cook for about 5 minutes, stirring often, until onion is softened.

Add flour. Heat and stir for 1 minute. Slowly add milk, stirring constantly, until smooth. Heat and stir until boiling and thickened.

(continued on next page)

Chicken & Turkey

Add next 5 ingredients and turkey. Cook for about 2 minutes, stirring occasionally, until heated through. Add to spaghetti. Stir until coated.

Add lemon zest. Stir well. Makes about 7 cups (1.75 L). Serves 4.

1 serving: 494 Calories; 6.4 g Total Fat (2.9 g Mono, 1.7 g Poly, 0.7 g Sat); 47 mg Cholesterol; 69 g Carbohydrate; 8 g Fibre; 45 g Protein; 528 mg Sodium

Pictured on page 72.

Note: If turkey breast cutlets are not available, use boneless, skinless turkey breast and cut into thin strips.

Devilled Turkey Meatballs

Tender turkey meatballs in a mildly sweet-and-sour sauce make a heavenly dish—with a kick of devilish heat!

Egg white (large), fork-beaten	1	1
Grated zucchini (with peel), squeezed dry	3/4 cup	175 mL
Fine dry bread crumbs	1/2 cup	125 mL
Grated onion	1/4 cup	60 mL
Sweet chili sauce	1 tbsp.	15 mL
Salt	1/4 tsp.	1 mL
Pepper	1/2 tsp.	2 mL
Extra-lean ground turkey thigh	3/4 lb.	340 g
Prepared chicken broth	1/2 cup	125 mL
Ketchup	3 tbsp.	50 mL
Sweet chili sauce	2 tbsp.	30 mL
Dijon mustard	1 tsp.	5 mL

Preheat oven to 400°F (205°C). Combine first 7 ingredients in medium bowl.

Add turkey. Mix well. Roll into balls, using about 1 tbsp. (15 mL) for each. Arrange in single layer on greased baking sheet with sides. Bake for about 15 minutes until fully cooked and internal temperature reaches 175°F (80°C).

Meanwhile, combine remaining 4 ingredients in large saucepan. Bring to a boil. Reduce heat to medium. Add meatballs. Heat and stir until meatballs are coated. Serves 4.

1 serving: 173 Calories; 2.2 g Total Fat (0.4 g Mono, 0.2 g Poly, 0.2 g Sat); 34 mg Cholesterol; 16 g Carbohydrate; 1 g Fibre; 24 g Protein; 665 mg Sodium

Cherry Turkey

*Tangy bites of dried cherries in a sweet maple sauce provide
the perfect accompaniment to turkey. Try using dried cranberries
if you can't find dried cherries at your supermarket.*

All-purpose flour	1/3 cup	75 mL
Salt	1/4 tsp.	1 mL
Pepper	1/4 tsp.	1 mL
Turkey breast scallopini (cut into 8 equal portions)	1 lb.	454 g
Olive (or canola) oil	1 1/2 tbsp.	25 mL
Olive (or canola) oil	1 tsp.	5 mL
Diced red onion	1 cup	250 mL
Prepared chicken broth	1/2 cup	125 mL
Dried cherries, chopped	1/3 cup	75 mL
Cherry jam	1/4 cup	60 mL
Maple (or maple-flavoured) syrup	3 tbsp.	50 mL
Balsamic vinegar	1 tbsp.	15 mL
Dried thyme	1/4 tsp.	1 mL

Combine first 3 ingredients on large plate. Press both sides of turkey into flour mixture until coated. Discard any remaining flour mixture.

Heat first amount of olive oil in large frying pan on medium-high. Cook turkey in 3 or 4 batches, for about 1 minute per side, until golden. Transfer to large plate. Cover to keep warm. Reduce heat to medium.

Add second amount of olive oil to same frying pan. Add onion. Cook for 3 to 5 minutes, stirring often, until onion starts to soften.

Add remaining 6 ingredients. Bring to a boil on medium. Cook for about 5 minutes, stirring occasionally, until sauce is reduced by half. Pour over turkey. Serves 4.

1 serving: 343 Calories; 7.9 g Total Fat (4.6 g Mono, 0.6 g Poly, 0.9 g Sat); 45 mg Cholesterol; 40 g Carbohydrate; 2 g Fibre; 30 g Protein; 329 mg Sodium

Ginger Sherry Salmon

With a stronger flavour than ginger ale, alcohol-free ginger beer (found in the import section of larger grocery stores) adds a tang to this recipe without the added heat of real ginger.

Bottle of ginger beer (alcohol-free)	10 1/2 oz.	296 mL
Dry sherry	1/4 cup	60 mL
Fresh (or frozen, thawed) salmon fillets (4 – 5 oz., 113 – 140 g, each), skin removed	4	4
Soy sauce	1 tbsp.	15 mL
Cornstarch	2 tsp.	10 mL
Chopped fresh parsley	2 tsp.	10 mL
Sesame seeds, toasted (see Tip, page 149), optional	2 tsp.	10 mL

Combine ginger beer and sherry in medium frying pan. Bring to a boil. Reduce heat to medium-low.

Add fillets. Simmer, covered, for 10 to 15 minutes until fish flakes easily when tested with fork. Transfer fillets to serving platter. Cover to keep warm. Strain ginger beer mixture into small saucepan. Discard solids. Bring to a boil. Reduce heat to medium. Boil gently, uncovered, for about 5 minutes until slightly reduced.

Stir soy sauce into cornstarch in small cup. Add to ginger beer mixture. Heat and stir until boiling and thickened. Pour over fillets.

Sprinkle with parsley and sesame seeds. Serves 4.

1 serving: 194 Calories; 7.2 g Total Fat (2.4 g Mono, 2.9 g Poly, 1.1 g Sat); 62 mg Cholesterol; 5 g Carbohydrate; trace Fibre; 23 g Protein; 251 mg Sodium

Pictured on page 126.

Steamed Mussel Bowls

A hint of fennel gives this dish its true "mussel."

Mussels	2 lbs.	900 g
Can of diced tomatoes, drained	14 oz.	398 mL
Dry (or alcohol-free) white wine	1/4 cup	60 mL
Prepared vegetable broth	1/4 cup	60 mL
Garlic cloves, minced	2	2
(or 1/2 tsp., 2 mL, powder)		
Fennel seed	1/4 tsp.	1 mL
Pepper	1/4 tsp.	1 mL
Sliced green onion	3 tbsp.	50 mL

Put mussels into medium bowl. Lightly tap to close any that are opened 1/4 inch (6 mm) or more (see Note). Discard any that do not close. Set aside.

Combine next 6 ingredients in Dutch oven. Bring to a boil. Reduce heat to medium.

Add green onion and mussels. Boil gently, covered, for about 8 minutes, without stirring, until mussels are opened. Transfer mussels with slotted spoon to 2 small serving bowls. Discard any unopened mussels. Ladle tomato mixture over mussels. Serves 2.

1 serving: 162 Calories; 2.7 g Total Fat (0.6 g Mono, 0.7 g Poly, 0.5 g Sat); 32 mg Cholesterol; 15 g Carbohydrate; trace Fibre; 16 g Protein; 925 mg Sodium

Note: For safety reasons, it is important to discard any mussels that do not close before cooking, as well as any that have not opened during cooking.

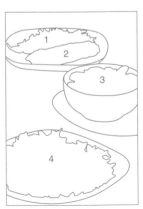

1. Lemony Carrot Salad, page 49
2. Chili-Rubbed Flank Steak, page 61
3. Orange Chili Beef, page 60
4. Beef And Sweet Potato Ragout, page 59

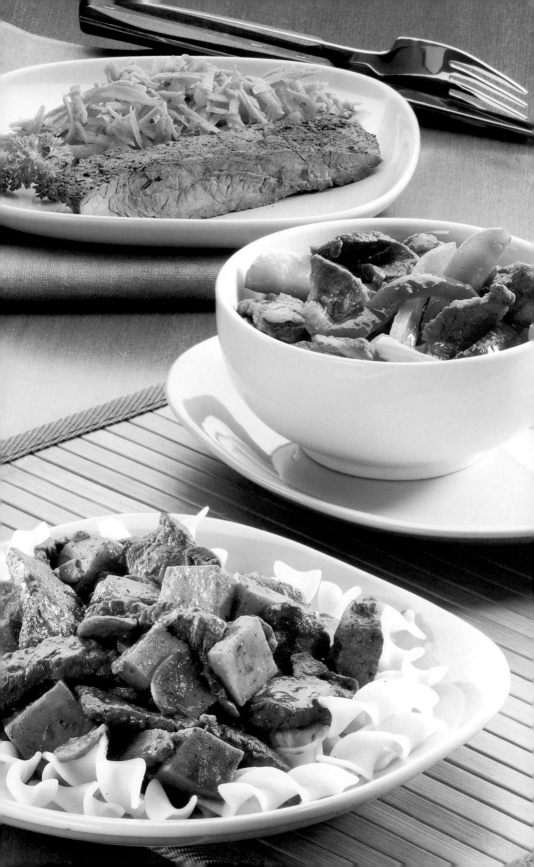

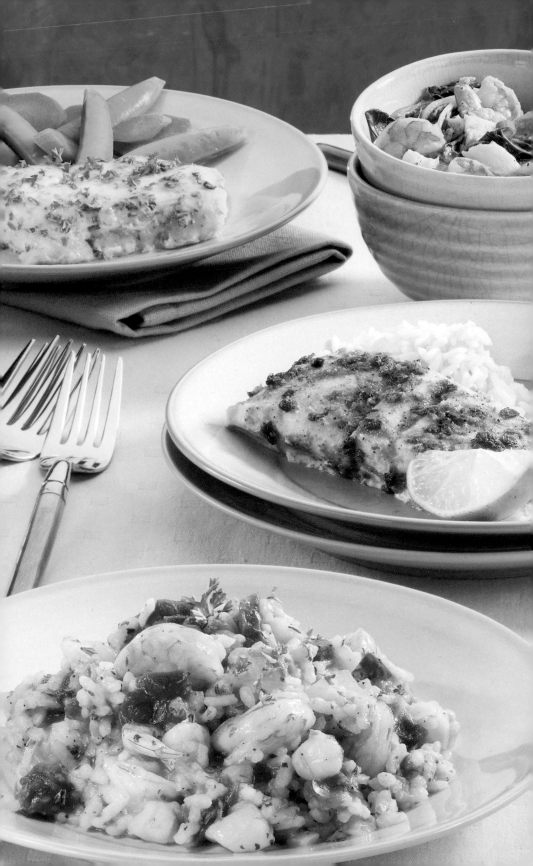

Baked Chipotle Halibut

Sweet spices and lime take halibut to a new taste level. Low in calories,
quick to prepare and off the Richter scale in taste.

Brown sugar, packed	2 tsp.	10 mL
Finely chopped chipotle pepper	2 tsp.	10 mL
in adobo sauce (see Tip, page 26)		
Garlic powder	1 tsp.	5 mL
Grated lime zest	1 tsp.	5 mL
Ground cumin	1/4 tsp.	1 mL
Salt	1/2 tsp.	2 mL
Pepper	1/8 tsp.	0.5 mL
Halibut fillets, any small bones removed	4	4
(4 – 5 oz., 113 – 140 g, each)		
Lime wedges, for garnish		

Preheat oven to 400°F (205°C). Combine first 7 ingredients in small cup.

Arrange fillets on baking sheet with sides, lined with greased foil. Spread brown sugar mixture evenly over fillets. Bake for 10 to 12 minutes until fish flakes easily when tested with fork.

Garnish with lime wedges. Serves 4.

1 serving: 138 Calories; 2.7 g Total Fat (0.9 g Mono, 0.8 g Poly, 0.4 g Sat); 36 mg Cholesterol; 3 g Carbohydrate; trace Fibre; 24 g Protein; 366 mg Sodium

Pictured at left.

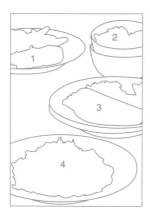

1. Tarragon Dijon Cod, page 98
2. Seafood Hotpot, page 94
3. Baked Chipotle Halibut, above
4. Seafood Risotto, page 92

Props courtesy of: Winners Stores

Seafood Risotto

An easy-to-make risotto with a taste like you've fussed for hours.
Shrimp and scallops are the perfect additions for that gourmet touch.

Prepared vegetable broth	2 1/2 cups	625 mL
Canola oil	1 tsp.	5 mL
Chopped onion	1 cup	250 mL
Arborio rice	1 cup	250 mL
Dry (or alcohol-free) white wine	1/4 cup	60 mL
Garlic cloves, minced	2	2
(or 1/2 tsp., 2 mL, powder)		
Dried basil	1 tsp.	5 mL
Dried oregano	1/2 tsp.	2 mL
Pepper	1/4 tsp.	1 mL
Can of diced tomatoes (with juice)	14 oz.	398 mL
Chopped fresh parsley	2 tbsp.	30 mL
(or 1 1/2 tsp., 7 mL, flakes)		
Lemon juice	1 tbsp.	15 mL
Granulated sugar	1/2 tsp.	2 mL
Prepared vegetable broth	1/4 cup	60 mL
Fresh (or frozen, thawed) small bay scallops	6 oz.	170 g
Frozen, uncooked medium shrimp	6 oz.	170 g
(peeled and deveined), thawed		
Chopped fresh parsley, for garnish		

Measure first amount of broth into medium saucepan. Bring to a boil. Reduce heat to low. Cover to keep hot.

Meanwhile, heat canola oil in large saucepan on medium-high. Add onion. Cook for 2 to 4 minutes, stirring often, until onion is softened.

Add next 6 ingredients. Heat and stir for about 1 minute until liquid is absorbed. Add hot broth. Bring to a boil. Reduce heat to medium-low. Simmer, covered, for about 15 minutes, without stirring, until rice is tender but firm and mixture is creamy.

Add next 4 ingredients. Stir.

(continued on next page)

Fish & Seafood

Meanwhile, measure second amount of broth into small saucepan. Bring to a boil. Reduce heat to medium. Add scallops and shrimp. Simmer, uncovered, for about 2 minutes, stirring occasionally, until scallops are opaque and shrimp turn pink. Drain. Add to rice mixture. Stir.

Garnish with parsley. Makes about 6 cups (1.5 L). Serves 4.

1 serving: 352 Calories; 3.2 g Total Fat (0.8 g Mono, 0.8 g Poly, 0.3 g Sat); 79 mg Cholesterol; 60 g Carbohydrate; 3 g Fibre; 22 g Protein; 693 mg Sodium

Pictured on page 90.

Thai Curry Fish Cakes

A taste of Thailand is readily apparent in our exotic fish cakes.
Packed with flavour, the red curry paste adds just the right zip!

White bread slices, crusts removed	2	2
Cod fillets, any small bones removed, chopped	1 lb.	454 g
Chopped green onion	1/4 cup	60 mL
Egg white (large)	1	1
Brown sugar, packed	1 tbsp.	15 mL
Garlic cloves, minced (or 1/2 tsp., 2 mL, powder)	2	2
Sesame oil (for flavour)	1 1/2 tsp.	7 mL
Finely grated gingerroot	1 tsp.	5 mL
Grated lime zest	1 tsp.	5 mL
Red curry paste	1 tsp.	5 mL
Chopped fresh basil	2 tbsp.	30 mL

Put bread slices into food processor. Process until broken up into crumbs. Transfer to small bowl.

Put next 9 ingredients into food processor. Process with on/off motion until combined.

Add basil and bread crumbs. Process with on/off motion until combined. Preheat broiler. Divide fish mixture into 12 equal portions. Shape into 1/2 inch (12 mm) thick patties. Arrange on greased baking sheet or broiler pan. Broil on top rack in oven for about 8 minutes until golden and firm. Immediately transfer patties to plate. Serves 4.

1 serving: 166 Calories; 3.2 g Total Fat (0.9 g Mono, 1.2 g Poly, 0.5 g Sat); 49 mg Cholesterol; 11 g Carbohydrate; trace Fibre; 22 g Protein; 187

Seafood Hotpot

Your house will become the dinner hotspot with this steamy delight.
Brimming with seaside goodness, this dish is great with rice or noodles.

Frozen, uncooked medium shrimp (peeled and deveined), thawed	1/2 lb.	225 g
Haddock fillets, any small bones removed, cut into bite-sized pieces	1/2 lb.	225 g
Fresh (or frozen, thawed) small bay scallops	1/4 lb.	113 g
Sesame oil (for flavour)	1 tsp.	5 mL
Garlic powder	1/2 tsp.	2 mL
Dried crushed chilies	1/4 tsp.	1 mL
Salt	1/4 tsp.	1 mL
Pepper	1/4 tsp.	1 mL
Prepared chicken broth	1 1/2 cups	375 mL
Gingerroot slices (1/4 inch, 6 mm, thick)	3	3
Soy sauce	1 tbsp.	15 mL
Star anise	1	1
Whole baby bok choy, halved lengthwise	5	5
Water	2 tbsp.	30 mL
Cornstarch	1 tbsp.	15 mL
Chopped green onion	1 tbsp.	15 mL

Combine first 8 ingredients in medium bowl. Set aside.

Combine next 4 ingredients in medium saucepan. Bring to a boil. Reduce heat to medium. Boil gently, covered, for 5 minutes to blend flavours.

Add bok choy. Simmer, covered, for about 5 minutes until almost tender-crisp. Add seafood mixture. Cook for about 1 minute until shrimp start to turn pink. Remove and discard ginger and anise.

Stir water into cornstarch in small cup. Add to seafood mixture. Stir. Cook, covered, for about 2 minutes until boiling and thickened and shrimp turn pink.

Add green onion. Stir. Makes about 4 cups (1 L). Serves 4.

1 serving: 168 Calories; 3.2 g Total Fat (0.8 g Mono, 1.2 g Poly, 0.6 g Sat); 128 mg Cholesterol; 5 g Carbohydrate; trace Fibre; 28 g Protein; 1080 mg Sodium

Pictured on page 90.

Shrimp Salmon Pasta

Just a bit of smoked salmon gives this recipe a rich taste that
makes a splash with the nutty flavour of whole wheat pasta.

Water	12 cups	3 L
Salt	1 1/2 tsp.	7 mL
Whole-wheat linguine	12 oz.	340 g
Prepared chicken broth	2/3 cup	150 mL
Dijon mustard	1 tsp.	5 mL
Granulated sugar	1 tsp.	5 mL
Dried dillweed	1/2 tsp.	2 mL
Garlic powder	1/4 tsp.	1 mL
Frozen, uncooked large shrimp (peeled and deveined), thawed	1/2 lb.	225 g
Water	1 tbsp.	15 mL
Cornstarch	1 tsp.	5 mL
Smoked salmon, cut into 1/4 inch (6 mm) strips	2 oz.	57 g
Evaporated milk (or half-and-half cream)	2 tbsp.	30 mL
Dried dillweed	1/4 tsp.	1 mL
Lemon wedges (optional)	4	4

Combine water and salt in Dutch oven or large pot. Bring to a boil.
Add pasta. Boil, uncovered, for 9 to 11 minutes, stirring occasionally,
until tender but firm. Drain. Return to same pot. Cover to keep warm.

Meanwhile, combine next 5 ingredients in medium saucepan. Bring to
a boil on medium. Add shrimp. Stir. Cook, covered, for about 1 minute
until shrimp start to turn pink.

Stir water into cornstarch in small cup. Add to shrimp mixture. Heat and
stir until boiling and thickened. Remove from heat.

Add next 3 ingredients. Stir. Add to pasta. Toss until coated.

Squeeze lemon wedges over individual servings. Makes about 5 cups (1.25 L).
Serves 4.

*1 serving: 407 Calories; 7.2 g Total Fat (0.6 g Mono, 0.6 g Poly, 1.2 g Sat); 90 mg Cholesterol;
57 g Carbohydrate; 12 g Fibre; 28 g Protein; 490 mg Sodium*

Speedy Tuna Primavera

*Who says land and sea don't mix? Primavera (Italian for "spring style"),
in the form of mixed veggies, is the way to go with canned tuna.
Hot pepper sauce adds a zesty new dimension.*

Water	12 cups	3 L
Salt	1 1/2 tsp.	7 mL
Fettuccine	12 oz.	340 g
Frozen California mixed vegetables	5 cups	1.25 L
Water	1/4 cup	60 mL
2% evaporated milk	1 cup	250 mL
All-purpose flour	3 tbsp.	50 mL
Prepared vegetable broth	1 cup	250 mL
Hot pepper sauce	1 tsp.	5 mL
Dried basil	1/2 tsp.	2 mL
Salt	1/2 tsp.	2 mL
Can of solid white tuna in water, drained, broken into chunks	6 oz.	170 g
Grated Parmesan cheese	1/2 cup	125 mL

Combine water and salt in Dutch oven or large pot. Bring to a boil.
Add fettuccine. Boil, uncovered, for 11 to 13 minutes, stirring occasionally,
until tender but firm. Drain. Return to same pot. Cover to keep warm.

Meanwhile, combine vegetables and water in medium microwave-safe
bowl. Microwave, covered, on high (100%) for about 8 minutes until
vegetables are tender-crisp. Drain. Cover to keep warm.

Whisk evaporated milk into flour in medium saucepan until smooth.
Add next 4 ingredients. Heat and stir on medium for about 5 minutes
until boiling and thickened.

Add tuna and vegetables. Stir. Add to fettuccine. Toss until coated.
Transfer to serving bowl.

Sprinkle with cheese. Makes about 8 cups (2 L). Serves 4.

*1 serving: 604 Calories; 9.8 g Total Fat (0.7 g Mono, 0.7 g Poly, 1.5 g Sat); 52 mg Cholesterol;
97 g Carbohydrate; 6 g Fibre; 35 g Protein; 1131 mg Sodium*

Sole Lay-Abouts

Sweet bites of apricot aren't the sole reason you'll love this dish. The bulgur and creamy-tasting, lemony dill sauce will invigorate your palate.

Prepared chicken broth	1 1/2 cups	375 mL
Bulgur	1 cup	250 mL
Chopped dried apricot	1/3 cup	75 mL
Seasoned salt	1/4 tsp.	1 mL
Sole fillets, any small bones removed (4 – 5 oz., 113 – 140 g, each)	6	6
Can of 2% evaporated milk	13 1/2 oz.	385 mL
All-purpose flour	1 tbsp.	15 mL
Dried dillweed	1/2 tsp.	2 mL
Grated lemon zest	1/2 tsp.	2 mL
Pepper	1/4 tsp.	1 mL
Lemon juice	2 tsp.	10 mL
Chopped fresh parsley (or 3/4 tsp., 4 mL, flakes)	1 tbsp.	15 mL

Preheat oven to 450°F (230°C). Measure broth into medium saucepan. Bring to a boil. Add next 3 ingredients. Stir. Reduce heat to medium. Simmer, covered, for about 5 minutes, stirring occasionally, until liquid is almost absorbed. Transfer to 9 × 13 inch (22 × 33 cm) pan. Spread evenly.

Arrange fillets in single layer over bulgur mixture. Cover with foil. Bake for 10 to 12 minutes until fish flakes easily when tested with fork.

Meanwhile, whisk evaporated milk into flour in small saucepan until smooth. Add next 3 ingredients. Heat and stir on medium-high until boiling and slightly thickened.

Stir in lemon juice and parsley. Pour over fillets and bulgur mixture. Serves 6.

1 serving: 316 Calories; 3.8 g Total Fat (0.9 g Mono, 0.8 g Poly, 1.4 g Sat); 83 mg Cholesterol; 31 g Carbohydrate; 3 g Fibre; 39 g Protein; 641 mg Sodium

Salsa Baked Cod

Your friends and family will dance after tasting this saucy salsa cod.
With only four ingredients, it's a fast and healthy low-fat dinner.

Cod fillets, any small bones removed (4 – 5 oz., 113 – 140 g, each)	4	4
Pepper	1/8 tsp.	0.5 mL
Salsa	3/4 cup	175 mL
Chopped fresh cilantro or parsley	1 tbsp.	15 mL

Preheat oven to 400°F (205°C). Arrange fillets in single layer in greased 2 quart (2 L) shallow baking dish. Sprinkle with pepper.

Spoon salsa over top. Bake for 15 to 20 minutes until fish flakes easily when tested with fork. Transfer fillets to serving platter.

Sprinkle with cilantro. Serves 4.

1 serving: 195 Calories; 1.6 g Total Fat (0.2 g Mono, 0.6 g Poly, 0.3 g Sat); 95 mg Cholesterol; 3 g Carbohydrate; 1 g Fibre; 40 g Protein; 330 mg Sodium

Tarragon Dijon Cod

This could be one of the most swimmingly fine fish dinners you've ever had.
Mustard and tarragon marry perfectly in this delicate dish.

Dry (or alcohol-free) white wine	1 tbsp.	15 mL
Honey Dijon mustard	1 tbsp.	15 mL
Dried tarragon	1/2 tsp.	2 mL
Cod fillets, any small bones removed (4 – 5 oz., 113 – 140 g, each)	4	4
Chopped fresh parsley	1 tbsp.	15 mL

Preheat oven to 400°F (205°C). Combine first 3 ingredients in small bowl.

Arrange fillets on greased baking sheet with sides. Brush with wine mixture. Bake for about 15 minutes until fish flakes easily when tested with fork.

Sprinkle with parsley. Serves 4.

(continued on next page)

Fish & Seafood

1 serving: 199 Calories; 3.0 g Total Fat (0.2 g Mono, 0.5 g Poly, 0.4 g Sat); 96 mg Cholesterol; 1 g Carbohydrate; trace Fibre; 39 g Protein; 139 mg Sodium

Pictured on page 90.

Shrimp And Bean Hotpot

If you haven't "bean" trying new seafood recipes, this is the place to start! Shrimp and beans are uncommonly tasty together and good for you, too.

Prepared chicken broth	2 cups	500 mL
Sliced carrot	1 cup	250 mL
Garlic cloves, minced	2	2
(or 1/2 tsp., 2 mL, powder)		
Dried rosemary, crushed	1 1/2 tsp.	7 mL
Pepper	1/4 tsp.	1 mL
Can of diced tomatoes (with juice)	14 oz.	398 mL
Can of navy beans, rinsed and drained	14 oz.	398 mL
Parsley flakes	1 tbsp.	15 mL
Frozen, uncooked medium shrimp	1 lb.	454 g
(peeled and deveined), thawed		
Prepared chicken broth	3 tbsp.	50 mL
Cornstarch	2 tbsp.	30 mL

Combine first 5 ingredients in large saucepan. Bring to a boil. Reduce heat to medium. Boil gently, uncovered, for about 5 minutes until carrot starts to soften.

Add next 3 ingredients. Bring to a boil. Reduce heat to medium.

Add shrimp. Cook for about 2 minutes until shrimp turn pink.

Stir second amount of broth into cornstarch in small cup. Add to shrimp mixture. Heat and stir until boiling and thickened. Makes about 7 cups (1.75 L). Serves 4.

1 serving: 304 Calories; 3.2 g Total Fat (0.6 g Mono, 1.2 g Poly, 0.7 g Sat); 172 mg Cholesterol; 36 g Carbohydrate; 7 g Fibre; 33 g Protein; 1735 mg Sodium

Mediterranean Pasta

Always wanted to give Swiss chard a try? Well, this delightfully savoury, slightly spicy tomato pasta dish gives you the perfect opportunity.

Water	8 cups	2 L
Salt	1 tsp.	5 mL
Fusilli pasta	3 cups	750 mL
Olive (or canola) oil	1 tsp.	5 mL
Chopped onion	1 cup	250 mL
Garlic cloves, minced	2	2
(or 1/2 tsp., 2 mL, powder)		
Chopped Swiss chard, lightly packed	4 cups	1 L
Can of chunky tomatoes	19 oz.	540 mL
(with juice), chopped (see Note)		
Dried crushed chilies	1/2 tsp.	2 mL
Dry (or alcohol-free) white wine	1/4 cup	60 mL
Can of white kidney beans,	19 oz.	540 mL
rinsed and drained		
Grated light Parmesan cheese	1/2 cup	125 mL

Combine water and salt in Dutch oven. Bring to a boil. Add pasta. Boil, uncovered, for 7 to 9 minutes, stirring occasionally, until tender but firm. Drain. Return to same pot. Cover to keep warm.

Meanwhile, heat olive oil in large frying pan on medium. Add onion and garlic. Cook for 5 to 10 minutes, stirring often, until softened.

Add next 3 ingredients. Stir. Cook, covered, for about 5 minutes until chard ribs are tender.

Add wine. Stir. Simmer, uncovered, for about 5 minutes until liquid is reduced by half.

Add beans. Cook and stir until heated through. Add to pasta.

Add cheese. Toss until coated. Makes about 8 cups (2 L). Serves 4.

1 serving: 887 Calories; 10.0 g Total Fat (0.9 g Mono, 0.2 g Poly, 3.0 g Sat); 10 mg Cholesterol; 157 g Carbohydrate; 27 g Fibre; 37 g Protein; 960 mg Sodium

Note: Cut tomatoes with a paring knife or kitchen shears while still in the can.

Meatless

Broccoli Pasta

This pasta and broccoli dish isn't creamy like you'd expect. Instead, it is coated with a light but intense peppery orange sauce that's lovely on the lips.

Water	12 cups	3 L
Salt	1 1/2 tsp.	7 mL
Whole-wheat linguine	12 oz.	340 g
Broccoli florets	6 cups	1.5 L
Water	1/4 cup	60 mL
Olive (or canola) oil	2 tsp.	10 mL
Chopped onion	1/2 cup	125 mL
Garlic clove, minced	1	1
(or 1/4 tsp., 1 mL, powder)		
Orange juice	1/2 cup	125 mL
Prepared chicken broth	1/2 cup	125 mL
Cornstarch	2 tsp.	10 mL
Grated orange zest	2 tsp.	10 mL
Salt	1/2 tsp.	2 mL
Pepper	1/2 tsp.	2 mL

Combine water and salt in Dutch oven or large pot. Bring to a boil. Add pasta. Boil, uncovered, for 9 to 11 minutes, stirring occasionally, until tender but firm. Drain. Return to same pot. Cover to keep warm.

Meanwhile, put broccoli into large microwave-safe bowl. Pour water over top. Microwave, covered, on high (100%) for 6 to 8 minutes until broccoli is tender-crisp.

Heat olive oil in small frying pan on medium. Add onion. Cook for about 5 minutes, stirring often, until onion starts to brown. Add garlic. Heat and stir for about 1 minute until fragrant.

Combine remaining 6 ingredients in small bowl. Add to onion mixture. Heat and stir until boiling and thickened. Add broccoli. Stir. Add to pasta. Toss until coated. Makes about 8 cups (2 L). Serves 6.

1 serving: 263 Calories; 5.4 g Total Fat (1.2 g Mono, 0.3 g Poly, 0.8 g Sat); 0 mg Cholesterol; 45 g Carbohydrate; 10 g Fibre; 12 g Protein; 354 mg Sodium

Quickstep Tamale Pie

We call it quickstep, because you have to be light on your toes to get your fair share before it's all gone! The crunchy cornmeal topping and mildly spicy mixed bean and salsa base will have your taste buds dancing.

Can of kidney beans, rinsed and drained	14 oz.	398 mL
Can of refried beans	14 oz.	398 mL
Frozen kernel corn	1 cup	250 mL
Salsa	1 cup	250 mL
Chili powder	1 tbsp.	15 mL
Yellow cornmeal	3/4 cup	175 mL
All-purpose flour	1/2 cup	125 mL
Baking powder	1 1/2 tsp.	7 mL
Salt	1/2 tsp.	2 mL
1% buttermilk	3/4 cup	175 mL
Canola oil	1 tbsp.	15 mL
Liquid honey	2 tsp.	10 mL
Grated light sharp Cheddar cheese	1 cup	250 mL

Preheat oven to 425°F (220°C). Combine first 5 ingredients in ungreased 2 quart (2 L) shallow baking dish. Microwave, partially covered, on high (100%) for about 5 minutes until bubbling around edges. Stir.

Meanwhile, measure next 4 ingredients into medium bowl. Stir. Make a well in centre.

Combine next 3 ingredients in small bowl. Add to well. Stir until just moistened.

Sprinkle cheese over bean mixture. Pour cornmeal mixture over top. Spread evenly. Bake for about 20 minutes until golden and wooden pick inserted in centre comes out clean. Serves 6.

1 serving: 351 Calories; 7.7 g Total Fat (1.8 g Mono, 1.0 g Poly, 2.8 g Sat); 17 mg Cholesterol; 54 g Carbohydrate; 10 g Fibre; 18 g Protein; 939 mg Sodium

Meatless

Veg 'N' Bean Burritos

It's hard to believe these mega-hearty cheesy burritos are low in fat. Trust us, you just gotta taste them to believe it! Serve with salsa on the side.

Canola oil	2 tsp.	10 mL
Sliced fresh white mushrooms	1 1/2 cups	375 mL
Chopped onion	1 cup	250 mL
Chili powder	1 tbsp.	15 mL
Parsley flakes	1 tbsp.	15 mL
Garlic clove, minced	1	1
(or 1/4 tsp., 1 mL, powder)		
Ground cumin	1/2 tsp.	2 mL
Salt	1/4 tsp.	1 mL
Can of black beans, rinsed and drained	19 oz.	540 mL
Frozen kernel corn	1/2 cup	125 mL
95% fat-free spreadable cream cheese	3/4 cup	175 mL
Whole-wheat flour tortillas	6	6
(9 inch, 22 cm, diameter)		
Grated light sharp Cheddar cheese	1/2 cup	125 mL

Heat canola oil in large frying pan on medium-high. Add mushrooms and onion. Cook for about 5 minutes, stirring often, until onion is softened and liquid is evaporated.

Add next 5 ingredients. Heat and stir for about 1 minute until fragrant.

Add beans and corn. Cook and stir for about 1 minute until heated through. Add cream cheese. Heat and stir until combined.

Spoon about 1/2 cup (125 mL) bean mixture across centre of each tortilla. Fold in sides. Roll up from bottom to enclose filling. Place, seam-side down, in greased 9 x 13 inch (22 x 33 cm) baking dish.

Sprinkle Cheddar cheese over top. Broil on centre rack in oven for about 5 minutes until cheese is melted and tortillas are crisp. Serves 6.

1 serving: 271 Calories; 8.7 g Total Fat (1.0 g Mono, 0.6 g Poly, 2.4 g Sat); 7 mg Cholesterol; 37 g Carbohydrate; 6 g Fibre; 14 g Protein; 922 mg Sodium

Braised Mushroom Ragout

*Instead of beef, this delicious stew has three kinds of mushrooms
for rich flavour. You won't believe how hearty and filling
mushrooms can be. Serve with crusty whole-grain bread.*

Package of dried porcini mushrooms	3/4 oz.	22 g
Boiling water	1 cup	250 mL
Canola oil	1 tsp.	5 mL
Chopped onion	1 cup	250 mL
Garlic clove, minced	1	1
(or 1/4 tsp., 1 mL, powder)		
Sliced fresh white mushrooms	3 cups	750 mL
Sliced portobello mushrooms	2 cups	500 mL
Grated carrot	1/2 cup	125 mL
Salt	1/4 tsp.	1 mL
Pepper	1/8 tsp.	0.5 mL
Prepared vegetable broth	2 cups	500 mL
Cornstarch	1 tbsp.	15 mL
Dried thyme	1/2 tsp.	2 mL
Can of navy beans, rinsed and drained	14 oz.	398 mL
Box of frozen chopped spinach,	10 oz.	300 g
thawed and squeezed dry		

Put porcini mushrooms into small heatproof bowl. Add boiling water. Stir.
Let stand, covered, for about 5 minutes until softened. Drain. Chop. Set aside.

Meanwhile, heat canola oil in large frying pan on medium-high. Add onion
and garlic. Cook for 3 to 5 minutes, stirring often, until onion starts to soften.

Add next 5 ingredients and porcini mushrooms. Cook for 5 to 10 minutes,
stirring often, until carrot is tender-crisp.

Combine next 3 ingredients in small bowl. Add to mushroom mixture. Stir.

Add beans and spinach. Stir. Reduce heat to medium-low. Cook, covered,
for about 5 minutes until boiling and thickened. Makes about 6 cups (1.5 L).
Serves 4.

*1 serving: 225 Calories; 2.5 g Total Fat (0.8 g Mono, 0.8 g Poly, 0.3 g Sat); 0 mg Cholesterol;
39 g Carbohydrate; 11 g Fibre; 14 g Protein; 892 mg Sodium*

Meatless

Curry Chickpea Roll-Ups

These remarkable roll-ups are a healthier version
of a baked burrito with an Indo-Asian twist.

Can of crushed tomatoes	14 oz.	398 mL
Non-fat plain yogurt	1 cup	250 mL
Curry powder	2 tsp.	10 mL
Granulated sugar	2 tsp.	10 mL
Ground cumin	1/2 tsp.	2 mL
Salt	1/2 tsp.	2 mL
Pepper	1/4 tsp.	1 mL
Can of chickpeas (garbanzo beans), rinsed and drained	19 oz.	540 mL
Frozen kernel corn, thawed	2 cups	500 mL
Whole-wheat flour tortillas (9 inch, 22 cm, diameter)	6	6

Preheat oven to 400°F (205°C). Combine first 7 ingredients in small bowl. Transfer 1/2 cup (125 mL) to medium bowl. Set aside remaining tomato mixture.

Add chickpeas and corn to tomato mixture in medium bowl. Mix well.

Spread chickpea mixture along centre of each tortilla. Fold in sides. Roll up from bottom to enclose filling. Place, seam-side down, in greased 9 x 13 inch (22 x 33 cm) pan. Pour reserved tomato mixture over top. Bake for about 20 minutes until bubbling and heated through. Serves 6.

1 serving: 283 Calories; 6.8 g Total Fat (0.4 g Mono, 0.8 g Poly, 1.0 g Sat); 1 mg Cholesterol;
46 g Carbohydrate; 6 g Fibre; 10 g Protein; 637 mg Sodium

Focaccia Pizza Pie

*Using an herbed focaccia bread as a fresh alternative to pizza crust
ups the flavour of this lip-smackingly tangy treat.*

Herb focaccia bread (10 inch, 25 cm, diameter), halved horizontally	1	1
Light ricotta cheese	1/2 cup	125 mL
Dried crushed chilies	1/2 tsp.	2 mL
Sun-dried tomatoes, softened in boiling water for 10 minutes before chopping	1/3 cup	75 mL
Large tomato, sliced	1	1
Thinly sliced onion	1/4 cup	60 mL
Crumbled light feta cheese	1/3 cup	75 mL
Grated medium tofu, drained	1/2 cup	125 mL
Grated part-skim mozzarella cheese	1/2 cup	125 mL

Preheat broiler. Place focaccia halves, cut-side up, on ungreased baking sheet with sides.

Spread ricotta cheese on focaccia halves, leaving 1 inch (2.5 cm) border around edge. Sprinkle with chilies.

Sprinkle remaining 6 ingredients, in order given, over ricotta cheese. Broil on centre rack in oven for 6 to 8 minutes until cheese is bubbling and starting to turn golden. Let stand for 5 minutes. Cut each half into 6 wedges. Serves 6.

1 serving: 126 Calories; 4.9 g Total Fat (0.6 g Mono, 0.4 g Poly, 2.7 g Sat); 16 mg Cholesterol; 11 g Carbohydrate; 1 g Fibre; 10 g Protein; 365 mg Sodium

1. Hot Fudge Mondaes, page 135
2. Miracle Mashed Potatoes, page 120
3. Peppery Balsamic Steaks, page 62
4. Glazed Brussels Sprouts, page 120

Props courtesy of: Canhome Global
Casa Bugatti
Winners Stores

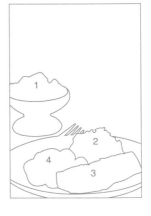

Meatless

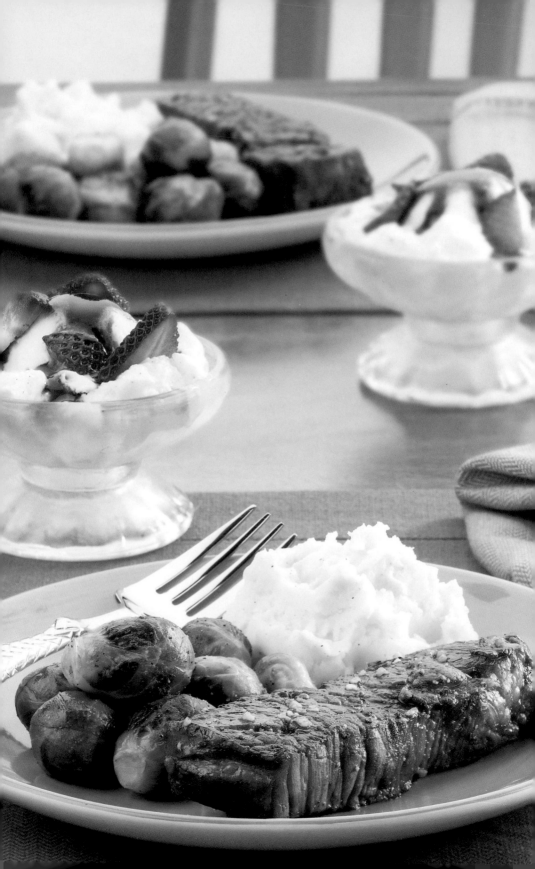

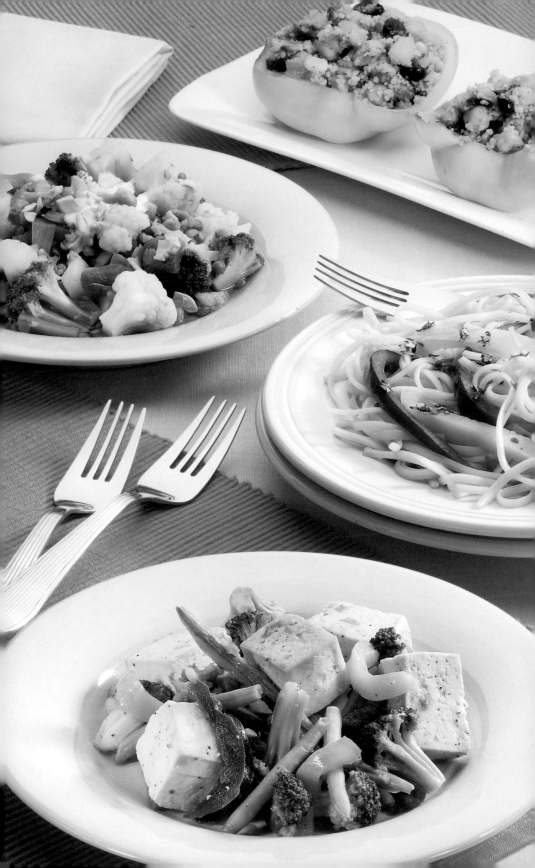

Honey Garlic Tofu

With lots of sweet and garlicky tofu, this vegetable
entree has plenty of flavour. Serve with rice.

Liquid honey	1/4 cup	60 mL
Apple juice	2 tbsp.	30 mL
Soy sauce	2 tbsp.	30 mL
Dijon mustard	1 tbsp.	15 mL
Garlic cloves, minced	3	3
(or 3/4 tsp., 4 mL, powder)		
Sesame oil (for flavour)	1/2 tsp.	2 mL
Pepper	1/4 tsp.	1 mL
Package of firm tofu, cut into	12 1/2 oz.	350 g
1 inch (2.5 cm) cubes		
Frozen Oriental mixed vegetables	6 cups	1.5 L

Combine first 7 ingredients in small bowl.

Heat large frying pan on medium. Add tofu and honey mixture. Cook and stir for about 5 minutes until heated through.

Add vegetables. Stir. Cook, covered, for 3 to 5 minutes until vegetables are tender-crisp. Makes about 6 cups (1.5 L). Serves 4.

1 serving: 263 Calories; 5.2 g Total Fat (0.7 g Mono, 1.6 g Poly, 0.9 g Sat); 1 mg Cholesterol;
41 g Carbohydrate; 1 g Fibre; 12 g Protein; 1319 mg Sodium

Pictured at left.

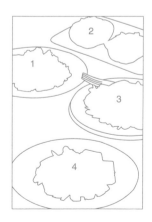

1. Vegetable Lentil Curry, page 111
2. Couscous Stuffed Peppers, page 110
3. Chili Linguine, page 112
4. Honey Garlic Tofu, above

Props courtesy of: Winners Stores

Couscous-Stuffed Peppers

Some see an empty bell pepper, we see a world of possibilities!
This time our vision includes curried whole-wheat couscous
flecked with cranberries and mushrooms.

Large yellow (or red) peppers, halved lengthwise	2	2
Prepared chicken broth	1 cup	250 mL
Whole-wheat couscous	1/2 cup	125 mL
Dried cranberries	1/3 cup	75 mL
Curry powder	1/2 tsp	2 mL
Ground cumin	1/4 tsp.	1 mL
Canola oil	1 tsp.	5 ml
Chopped onion	1/2 cup	125 mL
Sliced fresh white mushrooms	1/2 cup	125 mL
Garlic clove, minced (or 1/4 tsp., 1 mL, powder)	1	1
Canned chickpeas (garbanzo beans), rinsed and drained	1 cup	250 mL
Curry powder	1/2 tsp.	2 mL
Ground cumin	1/8 tsp.	0.5 mL
Salt	1/8 tsp.	0.5 mL
Pepper	1/8 tsp.	0.5 mL

Preheat oven to 450°F (230°C). Place yellow pepper halves, cut-side down, on greased baking sheet with sides. Bake for 12 to 15 minutes until tender-crisp.

Meanwhile, measure broth into medium saucepan. Bring to a boil. Add next 4 ingredients. Stir. Remove from heat. Let stand, covered, for about 5 minutes until liquid is absorbed. Fluff with fork. Cover to keep warm.

Heat canola oil in medium frying pan on medium. Add next 3 ingredients. Cook for about 5 minutes, stirring occasionally, until onion starts to soften.

Add remaining 5 ingredients. Stir. Cook, covered, for about 5 minutes until heated through. Add to couscous mixture. Stir well. Spoon into yellow pepper halves. Serves 4.

1 serving: 324 Calories; 5.1 g Total Fat (1.5 g Mono, 1.8 g Poly, 0.5 g Sat); 0 mg Cholesterol; 60 g Carbohydrate; 9 g Fibre; 14 g Protein; 461 mg Sodium

Pictured on page 108.

Vegetable Lentil Curry

*Cashews add a delightfully salty-sweet crunch
to this exquisite tomato-based lentil curry.*

Olive (or canola) oil	1 tsp.	5 mL
Chopped onion	1 1/2 cups	375 mL
Curry powder	2 tsp.	10 mL
Garlic clove, minced	1	1
(or 1/4 tsp., 1 mL, powder)		
Can of lentils, rinsed and drained	19 oz.	540 mL
Prepared vegetable broth	2 cups	500 mL
Can of diced tomatoes (with juice)	14 oz.	398 mL
Brown sugar, packed	2 tsp.	10 mL
Frozen California mixed vegetables	4 cups	1 L
Plain yogurt	1/3 cup	75 mL
Chopped salted cashews	1/4 cup	60 mL

Heat olive oil in Dutch oven on medium. Add next 3 ingredients. Cook for 5 to 10 minutes, stirring occasionally, until onion is softened.

Add next 4 ingredients. Stir. Bring to a boil. Reduce heat to medium-low. Add vegetables. Stir. Simmer, uncovered, for about 5 minutes until vegetables are tender-crisp. Transfer to large serving bowl.

Spoon yogurt over vegetable mixture. Sprinkle with cashews. Makes about 7 cups (1.75 L). Serves 4.

1 serving: 289 Calories; 7.0 g Total Fat (3.6 g Mono, 1.0 g Poly, 1.8 g Sat); 4 mg Cholesterol; 45 g Carbohydrate; 14 g Fibre; 14 g Protein; 762 mg Sodium

Pictured on page 108.

Paré Pointer

If at first you don't succeed...you'd better hope you aren't skydiving.

Chili Linguine

Explore new terrain with this unusual sweet-and-sour
pasta dish with a nice touch of heat.

Water	12 cups	3 L
Salt	1 1/2 tsp.	7 mL
Linguine	8 oz.	225 g
Brown sugar, packed	1/3 cup	75 mL
Apple cider vinegar	1/4 cup	60 mL
Soy sauce	2 tsp.	10 mL
Dried crushed chilies	1/2 tsp.	2 mL
Sesame oil (for flavour)	1/2 tsp.	2 mL
Sliced red pepper	1 cup	250 mL
Sliced yellow pepper	1 cup	250 mL
Chopped fresh cilantro or parsley	2 tsp.	10 mL

Combine water and salt in Dutch oven or large pot. Bring to a boil.
Add pasta. Boil, uncovered, for 9 to 11 minutes, stirring occasionally,
until tender but firm. Drain. Return to same pot. Cover to keep warm.

Combine next 5 ingredients in medium saucepan. Cook, uncovered,
on medium for 5 minutes to blend flavours.

Add red and yellow pepper. Stir. Cook for 2 to 3 minutes until peppers
are tender-crisp. Add to pasta. Toss until coated.

Sprinkle cilantro over top. Makes about 6 cups (2 L). Serves 4.

1 serving: 305 Calories; 1.6 g Total Fat (0.2 g Mono, 0.4 g Poly, 0.4 g Sat); trace Cholesterol;
66 g Carbohydrate; 3 g Fibre; 9 g Protein; 144 mg Sodium

Pictured on page 108.

Tomato Asparagus Pasta

*This creamy pasta dish has just enough gentle
heat to make you glow with satisfaction.*

Water	12 cups	3 L
Salt	1 1/2 tsp.	7 mL
Whole-wheat (or multi-grain) spaghetti	12 oz.	340 g
Olive (or canola) oil	1 tbsp.	15 mL
Garlic clove, minced	2	2
(or 1/2 tsp., 2 mL, powder)		
Dried crushed chilies	1/2 tsp.	2 mL
Can of chunky tomatoes (with juice)	19 oz.	540 mL
Fresh asparagus, trimmed of tough ends	2 cups	500 mL
and cut into 1 inch (2.5 cm) pieces		
Chopped sun-dried tomatoes	1/3 cup	75 mL
Light spreadable cream cheese	1/2 cup	125 mL

Combine water and salt in Dutch oven or large pot. Bring to a boil.
Add spaghetti. Boil, uncovered, for 10 to 12 minutes, stirring occasionally,
until tender but firm. Drain. Return to same pot. Cover to keep warm.

Heat olive oil in large frying pan on medium. Add garlic and chilies.
Heat and stir for about 1 minute until fragrant.

Add next 3 ingredients. Stir. Cook for about 5 minutes, stirring
occasionally, until asparagus is tender-crisp.

Add cream cheese. Stir until melted. Add to spaghetti. Stir until coated.
Makes about 7 cups (1.75 L). Serves 4.

*1 serving: 475 Calories; 9.7 g Total Fat (2.7 g Mono, 0.8 g Poly, 4.2 g Sat); 15 mg Cholesterol;
83 g Carbohydrate; 11 g Fibre; 19 g Protein; 840 mg Sodium*

Ginger Peas

Give your plain old peas a makeover with
a mix of gingery heat and smoky bacon.

Canola oil	1/2 tsp.	2 mL
Chopped onion	1 cup	250 mL
Finely grated gingerroot	1 tbsp.	15 mL
Garlic cloves, minced	2	2
(or 1/2 tsp., 2 mL, powder)		
Frozen peas	3 cups	750 mL
Prepared chicken broth	1/2 cup	125 mL
Salt	1/4 tsp.	1 mL
Pepper	1/4 tsp.	1 mL
Bacon bits	2 tbsp.	30 mL

Heat canola oil in medium saucepan on medium. Add next 3 ingredients. Cook for about 5 minutes, stirring occasionally, until onion starts to soften.

Add next 4 ingredients. Stir. Cook, covered, for about 5 minutes until peas are tender. Drain.

Sprinkle bacon bits over top. Makes about 3 cups (750 mL). Serves 4.

1 serving: 121 Calories; 1.7 g Total Fat (0.7 g Mono, 0.5 g Poly, 0.4 g Sat); 3 mg Cholesterol; 20 g Carbohydrate; 6 g Fibre; 7 g Protein; 381 mg Sodium

Cumin Mushrooms

These fried mushrooms take on a new taste with sour cream and are
the perfect accompaniment for a grilled steak and baked potato.

Halved fresh white mushrooms	4 cups	1 L
Prepared chicken broth	1/2 cup	125 mL
Garlic clove, minced	1	1
(or 1/4 tsp., 1 mL, powder)		
Ground cumin	1/2 tsp.	2 mL
Light sour cream	2 tbsp.	30 mL

(continued on next page)

Combine first 4 ingredients in large frying pan. Cook on medium-high for 15 to 20 minutes, stirring often, until mushrooms are tender and liquid is almost evaporated. Remove from heat.

Add sour cream. Stir. Makes about 2 cups (500 mL). Serves 4.

1 serving: 30 Calories; 0.9 g Total Fat (0.1 g Mono, 0.1 g Poly, 0.4 g Sat); 3 mg Cholesterol; 3 g Carbohydrate; trace Fibre; 2 g Protein; 196 mg Sodium

---

Curry-Sauced Cauliflower

This curried cauliflower dish with raisins, cashews and apple and orange flavours is simply stunning.

Curry powder	1 1/2 tsp.	7 mL
Apple juice	1/2 cup	125 mL
Orange juice	1/2 cup	125 mL
Raisins	1/2 cup	125 mL
Maple (or maple-flavoured) syrup	3 tbsp.	50 mL
Prepared mustard	1/2 tsp.	2 mL
Cauliflower florets	6 cups	1.5 L
Apple juice	1 tbsp.	15 mL
Cornstarch	2 tsp.	10 mL
Coarsely chopped salted cashews (optional)	2 tbsp.	30 mL

Heat large frying pan on medium-high. Add curry powder. Heat and stir for about 2 minutes until fragrant.

Add next 5 ingredients. Stir.

Add cauliflower. Stir. Bring to a boil. Reduce heat to medium. Boil gently, covered, for 5 to 10 minutes, stirring occasionally, until cauliflower is tender-crisp.

Stir second amount of apple juice into cornstarch in small cup. Add to cauliflower. Heat and stir until boiling and slightly thickened. Transfer to serving bowl.

Sprinkle cashews over top. Makes about 4 cups (1 L). Serves 4.

1 serving: 177 Calories; 0.5 g Total Fat (0.1 g Mono, 0.1 g Poly, 0.1 g Sat); 0 mg Cholesterol; 44 g Carbohydrate; 5 g Fibre; 4 g Protein; 60 mg Sodium

Sides

Spanish Rice

*Put a distinctive spin on a favourite side with
a little spice and lots of fresh veggies.*

Long grain white rice	1 cup	250 mL
Prepared vegetable (or chicken) broth	1 cup	250 mL
Water	3/4 cup	175 mL
Hot pepper sauce	1 tsp.	5 mL
Chili powder	1/2 tsp.	2 mL
Garlic powder	1/2 tsp.	2 mL
Paprika	1/2 tsp.	2 mL
Chopped tomato	1 cup	250 mL
Finely chopped green pepper	1/4 cup	60 mL
Chopped green onion	2 tbsp.	30 mL

Combine first 7 ingredients in large saucepan. Bring to a boil. Reduce heat to medium-low. Simmer, covered, for 15 minutes, without stirring. Remove from heat. Let stand, covered, for about 5 minutes until liquid is absorbed and rice is tender.

Add remaining 3 ingredients. Stir well. Makes about 5 cups (1.25 L). Serves 6.

1 serving: 138 Calories; 0.5 g Total Fat (0.1 g Mono, 0.1 g Poly, 0.1 g Sat); 0 mg Cholesterol; 30 g Carbohydrate; 1 g Fibre; 3 g Protein; 102 mg Sodium

Confetti Couscous

*This mix of olives, roasted red peppers, green onions and couscous makes any
meal a colourful celebration—but please, refrain from throwing this confetti!*

Low-sodium prepared chicken broth	1 3/4 cups	425 mL
Whole-wheat couscous	1 1/4 cup	300 mL
Dried oregano	1/2 tsp.	2 mL
Garlic powder	1/2 tsp.	2 mL
Light Italian dressing	2 tbsp.	30 mL
Diced roasted red pepper	3 tbsp.	50 mL
Chopped black olives	2 tbsp.	30 mL
Finely chopped green onion	2 tbsp.	30 mL

(continued on next page)

116 Sides

Measure broth into medium saucepan. Bring to a boil. Add next 3 ingredients. Stir. Remove from heat. Let stand, covered, for about 5 minutes until liquid is absorbed. Fluff with fork.

Add dressing. Toss.

Add remaining 3 ingredients. Stir. Makes about 4 cups (1 L). Serves 6.

1 serving: 112 Calories; 1.7 g Total Fat (0.2 g Mono, trace Poly, 0.3 g Sat); 2 mg Cholesterol; 21 g Carbohydrate; 3 g Fibre; 5 g Protein; 130 mg Sodium

Pictured on page 126.

Variation: Use light Greek dressing instead of Italian dressing.

Coconut Sweet Potato Mash

Sweet potatoes take an Asian holiday in this coconut and ginger-laden dish. Great with grilled chicken or pork.

Peeled orange-fleshed sweet potatoes, cubed	1 1/2 lbs.	680 g
GINGER COCONUT SAUCE		
Light coconut milk	1/2 cup	125 mL
Finely grated gingerroot	2 tsp.	10 mL
Garlic clove, minced (or 1/4 tsp., 1 mL, powder)	1	1
Dried crushed chilies (optional)	1/8 tsp.	0.5 mL
Lime juice	2 tsp.	10 mL
Salt	1/4 tsp.	1 mL

Pour water into large saucepan until about 1 inch (2.5 cm) deep. Add sweet potato. Cover. Bring to a boil. Reduce heat to medium. Boil gently for about 10 minutes until tender. Drain. Mash.

Ginger Coconut Sauce: Meanwhile, combine first 4 ingredients in small saucepan. Heat on medium for 5 minutes to blend flavours. Remove from heat.

Add lime juice and salt. Stir. Makes about 1/3 cup (75 mL) sauce. Add to mashed sweet potato. Stir well. Makes about 3 cups (750 mL). Serves 4.

1 serving: 207 Calories; 1.9 g Total Fat (0 g Mono, 0 g Poly, 1.4 g Sat); 0 mg Cholesterol; 43 g Carbohydrate; 5 g Fibre; 3 g Protein; 211 mg Sodium

Sides

Dilly Mashed Potatoes

*Perfect with salmon, this twist on mashed potatoes
has a subtle flavouring of fresh dill and lemon.*

Chopped peeled potato	5 cups	1.25 L
Skim milk	1/4 cup	60 mL
Chopped fresh dill	3 tbsp.	50 mL
(or 2 1/4 tsp., 11 mL, dried)		
Olive (or canola) oil	1 tbsp.	15 mL
Grated lemon zest	2 tsp.	10 mL
Salt	1/4 tsp.	1 mL

Pour water into large saucepan until about 1 inch (2.5 cm) deep. Add
potato. Cover. Bring to a boil. Reduce heat to medium. Boil gently for
12 to 15 minutes until tender. Drain. Mash.

Add remaining 5 ingredients. Mash. Makes about 4 cups (1 L). Serves 6.

*1 serving: 187 Calories; 2.5 g Total Fat (1.7 g Mono, 0.3 g Poly, 0.4 g Sat); trace Cholesterol;
39 g Carbohydrate; 4 g Fibre; 4 g Protein; 560 mg Sodium*

Broiled Sweet Potatoes

*This spicy and tangy chili orange glaze brings out the best in sweet potato.
Pair it perfectly with a savoury main course of chicken or fish.*

Medium peeled orange-fleshed	2 lbs.	900 g
sweet potatoes, cut into		
1/2 inch (12 mm) slices		
Water	1 tbsp.	15 mL
Sweet chili sauce	2 tbsp.	30 mL
Brown sugar, packed	1 tbsp.	15 mL
Orange juice	1 tbsp.	15 mL

Arrange sweet potato in single layer on microwave-safe plate. Sprinkle
with water. Microwave, covered, on high (100%) for about 5 minutes until
softened. Preheat broiler. Transfer sweet potato to broiler pan (see Note).

(continued on next page)

Sides

Combine remaining 3 ingredients in small cup. Brush over sweet potato. Broil on top rack in oven for 8 to 10 minutes until tender and browned. Serves 4.

1 serving: 261 Calories; 0.1 g Total Fat (0 g Mono, trace Poly, 0 g Sat); 0 mg Cholesterol; 60 g Carbohydrate; 7 g Fibre; 4 g Protein; 82 mg Sodium

Pictured on page 18.

Note: For easier cleanup, line the bottom of the broiler pan with foil. The sugary glaze can easily burn onto your pan.

Mustard Cream Leeks

Leeks are no longer a supporting player—when drizzled with a mustard wine cream sauce, they're certainly the star attraction! Great with salmon or pork.

Canola oil	1 tsp.	5 mL
Leeks (white part only), about 6 inches (15 cm) each, halved lengthwise	4	4
Prepared chicken broth	1 cup	250 mL
Dry (or alcohol-free) white wine	1/2 cup	125 mL
2% evaporated milk	1/2 cup	125 mL
Dijon mustard	1 tbsp.	15 mL
Garlic powder	1/4 tsp.	1 mL
Salt	1/4 tsp.	1 mL
Pepper	1/4 tsp.	1 mL

Heat canola oil in large frying pan on medium-high. Arrange half of leeks in frying pan. Cook for about 1 minute per side until browned. Transfer to plate. Repeat with remaining leeks.

Add broth and wine to same frying pan. Bring to a boil. Reduce heat to medium. Add leeks. Boil gently, covered, for 10 to 15 minutes until leeks are tender. Carefully transfer leeks with slotted spoon to serving platter. Cover to keep warm. Bring liquid in frying pan to a boil. Reduce heat to medium.

Add remaining 5 ingredients. Stir. Boil gently, uncovered, for 2 to 4 minutes until slightly thickened. Pour over leeks. Serves 4.

1 serving: 120 Calories; 2.3 g Total Fat (1.0 g Mono, 0.6 g Poly, 0.6 g Sat); 2 mg Cholesterol; 17 g Carbohydrate; 2 g Fibre; 4 g Protein; 620 mg Sodium

Glazed Brussels Sprouts

Put that cheese sauce away! A sweet and tangy balsamic glaze
is what really showcases beautifully roasted Brussels.

Frozen Brussels sprouts	4 cups	1 L
Olive oil	1 tbsp.	15 mL
Salt	1/2 tsp.	2 mL
Pepper	1/2 tsp.	2 mL
Balsamic vinegar	3 tbsp.	50 mL
Maple (or maple-flavoured) syrup	3 tbsp.	50 mL

Preheat oven to 425°F (220°C). Arrange Brussels sprouts on baking sheet with sides, lined with greased foil. Drizzle with olive oil. Toss until coated. Sprinkle with salt and pepper. Bake for about 20 minutes until tender. Transfer to serving bowl.

Combine vinegar and syrup in small cup. Drizzle over Brussels sprouts. Toss until coated. Makes about 3 cups (750 mL). Serves 4.

1 serving: 171 Calories; 4.4 g Total Fat (2.6 g Mono, 0.8 g Poly, 0.7 g Sat); 0 mg Cholesterol; 30 g Carbohydrate; 8 g Fibre; 9 g Protein; 321 mg Sodium

Pictured on page 107.

Miracle Mashed Potatoes

A little low-fat cream cheese can keep mashed potatoes
on your most-loved list without the added fat.

Chopped peeled potato	4 cups	1 L
Prepared chicken broth	1/3 cup	75 mL
Light cream cheese, softened	2 tbsp.	30 mL
Onion powder	1/2 tsp.	2 mL
Pepper	1/8 tsp.	0.5 mL

Pour water into large saucepan until about 1 inch (2.5 cm) deep. Add potato. Cover. Bring to a boil. Reduce heat to medium. Boil gently for 12 to 15 minutes until tender. Drain. Mash.

Add remaining 4 ingredients. Mash. Makes about 4 cups (1 L). Serves 4.

(continued on next page)

1 serving: 216 Calories; 1.6 g Total Fat (trace Mono, 0.1 g Poly, 1.0 g Sat); 4 mg Cholesterol; 46 g Carbohydrate; 5 g Fibre; 5 g Protein; 710 mg Sodium

Pictured on page 107.

Variation: Try a flavoured light cream cheese such as herb and garlic.

Fennel Apple Gratin

This fantastically sweet and savoury apple side with its golden crumb topping makes a fabulous flavour replacement for scalloped potatoes. Fuji or Golden Delicious apples work best for this recipe.

Canola oil	1 tsp.	5 mL
Sliced fennel bulb (white part only)	3 cups	750 mL
Prepared vegetable broth	1 cup	250 mL
Dried basil	1/2 tsp.	2 mL
Garlic powder	1/4 tsp.	1 mL
Salt	1/4 tsp.	1 mL
Pepper	1/4 tsp.	1 mL
Sliced peeled apple	2 cups	500 mL
Fine dry bread crumbs	1/2 cup	125 mL
Grated Parmesan cheese	1/4 cup	60 mL
Parsley flakes	2 tsp.	10 mL
Butter (or hard margarine), melted	1 tsp.	5 mL

Heat canola oil in large frying pan on medium. Add fennel. Cook for about 5 minutes, stirring occasionally, until fennel starts to soften.

Add next 5 ingredients. Stir. Bring to a boil. Reduce heat to medium. Boil gently, covered, for 5 minutes.

Add apple. Stir. Cook, uncovered, for 2 to 4 minutes until fennel is tender-crisp and liquid is almost evaporated.

Preheat broiler. Combine remaining 4 ingredients in small bowl. Sprinkle over fennel mixture. Broil on centre rack in oven for about 4 minutes (see Tip, page 22) until golden. Makes about 5 cups (1.25 L). Serves 6.

1 serving: 221 Calories; 8.5 g Total Fat (2.8 g Mono, 0.5 g Poly, 4.4 g Sat); 18 mg Cholesterol; 27 g Carbohydrate; 7 g Fibre; 12 g Protein; 729 mg Sodium

Hot Chili Quinoa

*Healthy quinoa (pronounced KEEN-wah) is finally coming
into its own in this side dish that has it all—sweetness, spice and
a texture that can't be beat. Great with grilled chicken or pork.*

Prepared vegetable broth	1 1/2 cups	375 mL
Quinoa, rinsed and drained	1 cup	250 mL
Canola oil	1 tsp.	5 mL
Chopped onion	1 cup	250 mL
Garlic clove, minced	1	1
(or 1/4 tsp., 1 mL, powder)		
Chopped green pepper	1/2 cup	125 mL
Sun-dried tomatoes, softened in boiling	1/2 cup	125 mL
water for 10 minutes before chopping		
Finely diced fresh hot chili pepper	1 tbsp.	15 mL
(see Tip, page 26)		
Balsamic vinegar	3 tbsp.	50 mL
Liquid honey	2 tbsp.	30 mL
Pepper	1/4 tsp.	1 mL
Pine nuts, toasted (see Tip, page 149)	1/4 cup	60 mL

Measure broth into medium saucepan. Bring to a boil. Add quinoa. Stir.
Reduce heat to medium-low. Simmer, covered, for about 20 minutes,
without stirring, until quinoa is tender and liquid is absorbed. Fluff with
fork. Cover to keep warm.

Meanwhile, heat canola oil in large pan on medium. Add onion and garlic.
Cook for 5 to 10 minutes, stirring often, until onion is softened.

Add next 3 ingredients. Stir. Cook for about 2 minutes, stirring
occasionally, until green pepper starts to soften. Add quinoa.

Combine next 3 ingredients in small cup. Drizzle over quinoa mixture.
Stir until coated.

Sprinkle pine nuts over top. Makes about 4 cups (1 L). Serves 4.

*1 serving: 319 Calories; 9.1 g Total Fat (3.3 g Mono, 3.6 g Poly, 1.2 g Sat); 0 mg Cholesterol;
52 g Carbohydrate; 7 g Fibre; 10 g Protein; 329 mg Sodium*

Pictured on page 125.

Lemon Ginger Pilaf

This quick and easy pilaf is loaded with whole-grain bulgur
and tender-crisp veggies. Chilies and ginger give it a real zing.

Prepared vegetable broth	2 cups	500 mL
Bulgur	1 1/2 cups	375 mL
Canola oil	1 tsp.	5 mL
Sliced fresh white mushrooms	2 cups	500 mL
Chopped onion	1 cup	250 mL
Chopped zucchini (with peel)	1 1/2 cups	375 mL
Chopped red pepper	1 cup	250 mL
Chopped yellow pepper	1 cup	250 ml
Liquid honey	1/4 cup	60 mL
Lemon juice	2 tbsp.	30 mL
Finely grated gingerroot	1 tbsp.	15 mL
Grated lemon zest	1 tsp.	5 mL
Garlic powder	1/2 tsp.	2 mL
Salt	1/4 tsp.	1 mL
Pepper	1/4 tsp.	1 mL
Dried crushed chilies	1/8 tsp.	0.5 mL

Measure broth into medium saucepan. Bring to a boil. Add bulgur. Stir.
Reduce heat to medium. Simmer, covered, for 8 minutes, without stirring.
Remove from heat. Let stand, covered, for about 10 minutes until liquid
is absorbed.

Meanwhile, heat canola oil in large frying pan on medium. Add
mushrooms and onion. Cook for about 5 minutes, stirring often,
until onion starts to soften.

Add remaining 11 ingredients. Stir. Cook for about 5 minutes, stirring
occasionally, until vegetables are tender-crisp. Transfer to large bowl.
Add bulgur. Stir well. Makes about 7 cups (1.75 L). Serves 6.

1 serving: 219 Calories; 1.6 g Total Fat (0.5 g Mono, 0.5 g Poly, trace Sat); 0 mg Cholesterol;
48 g Carbohydrate; 6 g Fibre; 6 g Protein; 263 mg Sodium

Pictured on page 125.

Balsamic Veggies

*This easy and colourful blend of balsamic veggies will add
simple elegance to any main. (If your asparagus stalks are
quite thick, cut them in half lengthwise before cooking.)*

Fresh asparagus, trimmed of tough ends	1 lb.	454 g
Sliced yellow pepper	1 cup	250 mL
Garlic clove, minced	1	1
(or 1/4 tsp., 1 mL, powder)		
Cherry tomatoes, halved	1 cup	250 mL
Balsamic vinegar	2 tbsp.	30 mL
Salt, sprinkle		
Pepper, sprinkle		
Chopped fresh basil (or parsley)	1 tbsp.	15 mL

Pour water into large frying pan until about 1 inch (2.5 cm) deep. Bring
to a boil. Reduce heat to medium. Add first 3 ingredients. Stir. Boil gently,
covered, for 3 to 5 minutes until asparagus is tender-crisp. Drain.

Add tomatoes. Heat and stir for about 2 minutes until tomatoes are hot.
Remove from heat.

Drizzle with balsamic vinegar. Sprinkle with salt and pepper. Stir.

Sprinkle basil over top. Serves 6.

*1 serving: 36 Calories; 0.1 g Total Fat (trace Mono, 0.1 g Poly, trace Sat); 0 mg Cholesterol;
7 g Carbohydrate; 2 g Fibre; 2 g Protein; 4 mg Sodium*

Pictured at right.

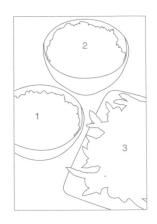

1. Hot Chili Quinoa, page 122
2. Lemon Ginger Pilaf, page 123
3. Balsamic Veggies, above

Props courtesy of: Danesco Inc.

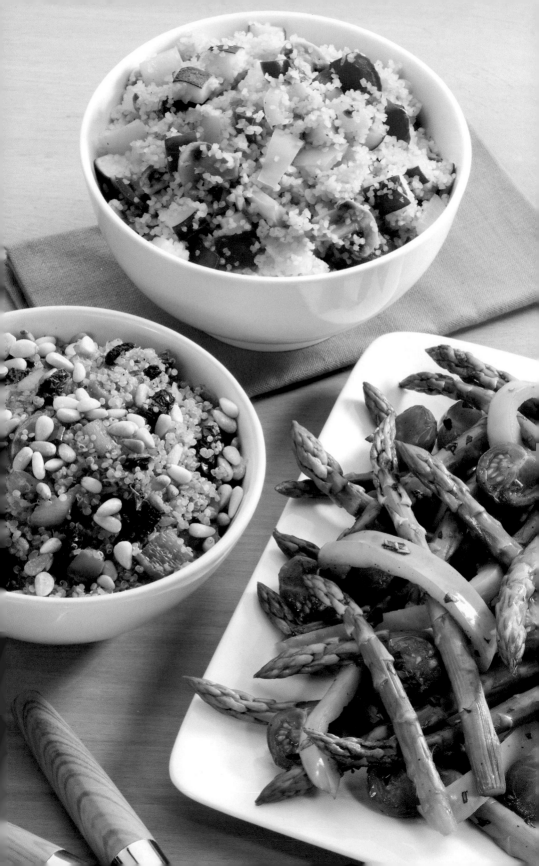

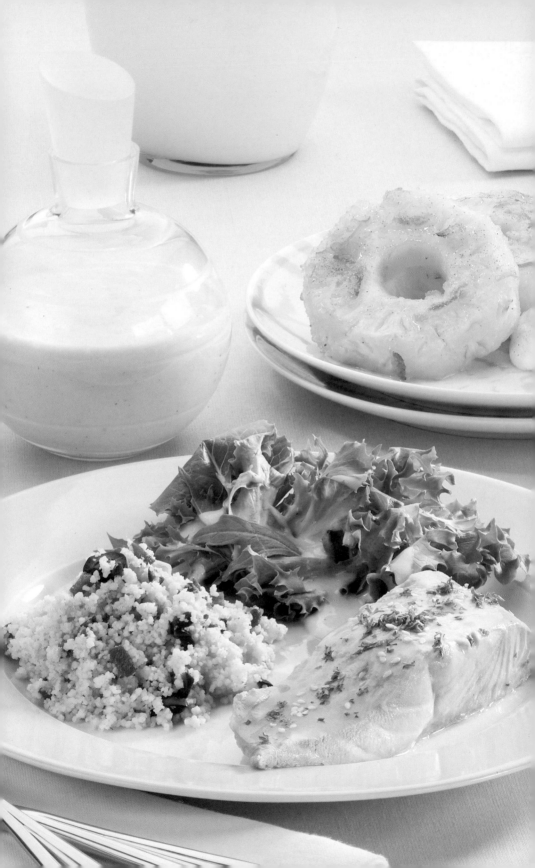

Mushroom Rice Pilaf

With lots of mushrooms, Parmesan cheese and Italian spices,
the flavours in this side are abundantly pleasing.

Sliced fresh white mushrooms	2 cups	500 mL
Fat-free Italian dressing	1/4 cup	60 mL
Water	1 1/2 cups	375 mL
Italian seasoning	1/2 tsp.	2 mL
Long grain white rice	1 cup	250 mL
Grated light Parmesan cheese	2 tbsp.	30 mL
Paprika	1/4 tsp.	1 mL

Heat medium frying pan on medium-high. Add mushrooms and dressing.
Cook for 3 to 4 minutes, stirring occasionally, until mushrooms are soft.

Meanwhile, combine water and Italian seasoning in medium saucepan.
Bring to a boil. Add rice and mushrooms. Stir. Reduce heat to medium-low.
Simmer, covered, for 15 minutes, without stirring. Remove from heat.
Let stand, covered, for about 5 minutes, until liquid is absorbed and
rice is tender.

Sprinkle with cheese. Fluff with fork. Sprinkle with paprika. Makes about
3 1/2 cups (875 mL). Serves 4.

1 serving: 249 Calories; 2.2 g Total Fat (0.1 g Mono, 0.1 g Poly, 0.2 g Sat); 7.6 mg Cholesterol;
49 g Carbohydrate; 1 g Fibre; 8 g Protein; 331 mg Sodium

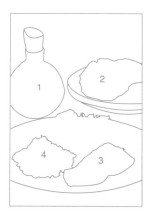

1. Mango Dressing, page 57
2. Broiled Pineapple, page 139
3. Ginger Sherry Salmon, page 87
4. Confetti Couscous, page 116

Props courtesy of: Casa Bugatti
Mikasa Home Store
Pier 1 Imports

Sides

Spinach Fettuccine

*Another creamy and flavourful side you just won't
believe is low fat. Thank the flavourful goat cheese for that!
For a milder flavour, use light cream cheese instead.*

Water	12 cups	3 L
Salt	1 1/2 tsp.	7 mL
Spinach fettuccine	12 oz.	340 g
Can of diced tomatoes (with juice)	14 oz.	398 mL
Prepared chicken broth	3/4 cup	175 mL
Garlic and herb no-salt seasoning	1 tsp.	5 mL
Soft goat (chèvre) cheese	1/3 cup	75 mL
(about 2 1/4 oz., 63 g), cut up		
Chopped fresh parsley	2 tbsp.	30 mL
(or 1 1/2 tsp., 7 mL, flakes)		
Coarsely ground pepper	1/8 tsp.	0.5 mL

Combine water and salt in Dutch oven or large pot. Bring to a boil.
Add fettuccine. Boil, uncovered, for 11 to 13 minutes, stirring occasionally,
until tender but firm. Drain, reserving 1/2 cup (125 mL) cooking water.
Return fettuccine to same pot. Cover to keep warm.

Meanwhile, combine next 3 ingredients in medium saucepan. Bring to
a boil. Pour over fettuccine.

Add remaining 3 ingredients. Toss, adding reserved cooking water a little
at a time, if needed, to moisten. Makes about 6 cups (1.5 L). Serves 6.

*1 serving: 232 Calories; 3.2 g Total Fat (0.7 g Mono, 0.9 g Poly, 1.5 g Sat); 4 mg Cholesterol;
43 g Carbohydrate; 2 g Fibre; 10 g Protein; 495 mg Sodium*

Paré Pointer

He thinks cartoons are what you listen to while driving.

Sides

Hot Pudding Cakes

These divine lava cakes have intriguing chocolate pudding centres.
No one would ever guess they're low in fat!

Bittersweet chocolate baking squares (1 oz., 28 g, each), coarsely chopped	2	2
Low-cholesterol egg product	3/4 cup	175 mL
Granulated sugar	2/3 cup	150 mL
Unsweetened applesauce	1/2 cup	125 mL
Canola oil	1 1/2 tbsp.	25 mL
Vanilla extract	1 tsp.	5 mL
Cocoa, sifted if lumpy	1/2 cup	125 mL
All-purpose flour	1/4 cup	60 mL
Salt	1/8 tsp.	0.5 mL

Preheat oven to 400°F (205°C). Put chocolate into medium microwave-safe bowl. Microwave, uncovered, on medium (50%) for about 90 seconds, stirring every 30 seconds, until almost melted (see Tip, below). Do not overheat. Stir until smooth.

Combine next 5 ingredients in small bowl. Slowly whisk egg mixture into melted chocolate until combined.

Combine remaining 3 ingredients in separate small bowl. Add to chocolate mixture. Whisk until combined. Spoon into 6 greased ramekins. Place ramekins on baking sheet with sides. Bake for 12 to 14 minutes until sides and top are set but wooden pick inserted in centre comes out wet with batter. Serve immediately. Serves 6.

1 serving: 225 Calories; 10.0 g Total Fat (4.0 g Mono, 1.2 g Poly, 3.8 g Sat); 26 mg Cholesterol; 34 g Carbohydrate; 4 g Fibre; 6 g Protein; 95 mg Sodium

Pictured on page 143.

 tip The microwaves used in our test kitchen are 900 watts—but microwaves are sold in many different powers. You should be able to find the wattage of yours by opening the door and looking for the mandatory label. Especially when microwaving chocolate, if your microwave is more than 900 watts, you may need to reduce the cooking time. If it's less than 900 watts, you'll probably need to increase the cooking time.

Desserts

Chocolate Crepes

Put a little of Paris on your plate with these quick and
easy-to-make chocolate crepes topped with sweet strawberry syrup.
Serve with frozen yogurt for some added flair.

TOPPING		
Container of frozen strawberries in light syrup	15 oz.	425 g
Water	2 tsp.	10 mL
Cornstarch	1 tbsp.	15 mL
CHOCOLATE CREPES		
All-purpose flour	3/4 cup	175 mL
Cocoa, sifted if lumpy	1/4 cup	60 mL
Granulated sugar	2 tbsp.	30 mL
Salt	1/2 tsp.	2 mL
Large eggs	3	3
Skim milk	1 1/4 cups	300 mL
Canola oil	1 tbsp.	15 mL

Topping: Heat strawberries with syrup in small saucepan on medium for 5 to 10 minutes, stirring occasionally, until heated through.

Stir water into cornstarch in small cup. Add to strawberries. Heat and stir until boiling and thickened. Remove from heat. Cover to keep warm.

Chocolate Crepes: Meanwhile, measure first 4 ingredients into medium bowl. Stir. Make a well in centre.

Whisk remaining 3 ingredients in small bowl until smooth. Add to well. Whisk until smooth. Makes about 2 1/2 cups (625 mL). Heat small (8 inch, 20 cm) non-stick frying pan on medium. Spray with cooking spray. Pour about 1/4 cup (60 mL) batter into frying pan. Immediately swirl to coat bottom of pan, lifting and tilting to coat entire bottom of pan. Cook until top is set and surface appears dry. Remove to plate. Fold into quarters. Repeat with remaining batter, spraying with cooking spray between batches. Makes about 10 crepes. Pour topping over crepes. Serves 4.

1 serving: 284 Calories; 8.0 g Total Fat (3.4 g Mono, 1.2 g Poly, 1.9 g Sat); 141 mg Cholesterol; 45 g Carbohydrate; 2 g Fibre; 11 g Protein; 380 mg Sodium

(continued on next page)

Pictured on page 143.

Variation: Fold each crepe around 1/2 cup (125 mL) non-fat frozen yogurt and top with syrup.

Blueberry Peach Crumble

Feeling blue? This bubbly blueberry bake is sure to lighten your mood. With sweet, juicy fruit and a buttery golden crumb topping, it only tastes like an indulgence.

FRUIT COMPOTE

Can of sliced peaches in juice (with juice)	14 oz.	398 mL
Fresh (or frozen) blueberries	1 cup	250 mL
Brown sugar, packed	2 tbsp.	30 mL
Minute tapioca	1 tsp.	5 mL

TOPPING

Butter (or hard margarine)	2 tbsp.	30mL
Quick-cooking rolled oats (not instant)	1/2 cup	125 mL
Brown sugar, packed	3 tbsp.	50 mL
Whole-wheat flour	2 tbsp.	30 mL

Fruit Compote: Preheat oven to 425°F (220°C). Combine all 4 ingredients in medium microwave-safe bowl. Microwave, uncovered, on high (100%) for about 5 minutes until boiling. Stir. Makes about 2 cups (500 mL) compote.

Topping: Meanwhile, melt butter in small saucepan on medium. Add remaining 3 ingredients. Stir until mixture resembles coarse crumbs. Spoon compote into 4 ramekins. Place ramekins on foil-lined baking sheet. Sprinkle topping over compote. Bake for about 10 minutes until tops are golden and filling is bubbling. Let stand for 5 minutes. Serves 4.

1 serving: 237 Calories; 6.7 g Total Fat (1.5 g Mono, 0.3 g Poly, 3.6 g Sat); 15 mg Cholesterol; 44 g Carbohydrate; 4 g Fibre; 3 g Protein; 52 mg Sodium

Pictured on page 143.

Chocolate Banana Bake

With its unique crumbly topping, this dessert is like a banana crisp with a delectable dose of chocolate. Best served warm.

Medium bananas, cut into 1 inch (2.5 cm) pieces	6	6
Lemon juice	2 tsp.	10 mL
Quick-cooking rolled oats (not instant)	1/2 cup	125 mL
All-purpose flour	1/4 cup	60 mL
Brown sugar, packed	1/4 cup	60 mL
Butter (or hard margarine), softened	2 tbsp.	30 mL
Semi-sweet chocolate chips	1/4 cup	60 mL

Preheat oven to 425°F (220°C). Put banana and lemon juice into medium bowl. Toss. Transfer to greased 2 quart (2 L) shallow baking dish.

Combine next 3 ingredients in small bowl.

Add butter. Rub between fingers until mixture resembles coarse crumbs. Add chocolate chips. Stir. Sprinkle over banana mixture. Bake for about 15 minutes until topping is browned and banana is tender. Makes about 5 cups (1.25 L). Serves 6.

1 serving: 251 Calories; 6.8 g Total Fat (1.7 g Mono, 0.3 g Poly, 3.8 g Sat); 10 mg Cholesterol; 49 g Carbohydrate; 4 g Fibre; 3 g Protein; 32 mg Sodium

Strawberry Whirl

This fluffy, mousse-style strawberry confection will leave you feeling as light as air. Serve immediately after preparing.

Box of strawberry jelly powder (gelatin)	3 oz.	85 g
Boiling water	3/4 cup	175 mL
Bag of frozen whole strawberries	24 oz.	600 g
95% fat-free spreadable cream cheese	1/2 cup	125 mL
Frozen light whipped topping, thawed	1 cup	250 mL

(continued on next page)

Put jelly powder and boiling water into food processor. Process until jelly powder is dissolved.

Slowly add strawberries, 1/2 cup (125 mL) at a time, processing after each addition until almost smooth. Add cream cheese. Process with on/off motion until combined. Transfer to large bowl.

Fold in whipped topping. Makes about 6 1/2 cups (1.6 L). Serves 6.

1 serving: 185 Calories; 1.8 g Total Fat (0.1 g Mono, 0.1 g Poly, 1.5 g Sat); 2 mg Cholesterol; 41 g Carbohydrate; 2 g Fibre; 5 g Protein; 164 mg Sodium

Tropical Pudding

Our melt-in-your-mouth version of the classic ambrosia salad would leave the gods themselves smiling.

Light sour cream	1 cup	250 mL
Reserved pineapple juice	1/2 cup	125 mL
Skim milk	1/2 cup	125 mL
Box of instant vanilla pudding powder (4-serving size)	1	1
Coconut extract	1 tsp.	5 mL
Ground ginger	1/4 tsp.	1 mL
Can of crushed pineapple, drained and juice reserved	14 oz.	398 mL
Miniature white marshmallows	1/2 cup	125 mL
Large banana, sliced	1	1
Medium sweetened coconut, toasted (see Tip, page 149)	2 tbsp.	30 mL
Sliced almonds, toasted (see Tip, page 149)	2 tbsp.	30 mL

Combine first 3 ingredients in large bowl.

Add next 3 ingredients. Whisk for about 2 minutes until combined and slightly fluffy.

Add next 3 ingredients. Stir well. Spoon into 4 small bowls.

Sprinkle coconut and almonds over top. Makes about 4 cups (1 L). Serves 4.

1 serving: 340 Calories; 8.6 g Total Fat (1.5 g Mono, 0.6 g Poly, 4.3 g Sat); 21 mg Cholesterol; 58 g Carbohydrate; 2 g Fibre; 6 g Protein; 439 mg Sodium

Apples 'N' Maple Cream

For a decadent delight that won't tip the scales, this maple-laced ricotta cream served over tart apple is both sinfully rich and angelically healthy!

Brown sugar, packed	2/3 cup	150 mL
Medium tart apples (such as Granny Smith), peeled and cut into 8 wedges each	4	4

MAPLE CREAM		
Light ricotta cheese	1 cup	250 mL
Maple (or maple-flavoured) syrup	1/4 cup	60 mL
Granulated sugar	1 tbsp.	15 mL
Dark (navy) rum (or 1/4 tsp., 1 mL, rum extract)	2 tsp.	10 mL

Heat large frying pan on medium. Sprinkle brown sugar over bottom of pan. Arrange apple in single layer over sugar. Cook for 8 to 10 minutes, turning at halftime, until apple is tender and brown sugar is syrupy.

Maple Cream: Meanwhile, put all 4 ingredients into blender. Process until smooth and light. Makes about 1 1/4 cups (300 mL) cream. Serve over apples. Serves 4.

1 serving: 327 Calories; 2.5 g Total Fat (trace Mono, trace Poly, 1.5 g Sat); 15 mg Cholesterol; 72 g Carbohydrate; 3 g Fibre; 5 g Protein; 72 mg Sodium

Pictured on page 18.

Five-Spice Mango

Dessert can be as easy as this—just a little five-spice powder lends a flavourful flair to mango.

Brown sugar, packed	3 tbsp.	50 mL
Butter (or hard margarine)	2 tbsp.	30 mL
Chinese five-spice powder	1/2 tsp.	2 mL
Frozen mango pieces	3 cups	750 mL
Lime sherbet	2 cups	500 mL

(continued on next page)

Combine first 3 ingredients in large frying pan. Heat on medium until bubbling and fragrant.

Add mango. Stir. Cook for 8 to 10 minutes, stirring occasionally, until heated through and syrupy. Let stand for 5 minutes.

Spoon sherbet into 4 small bowls. Spoon mango mixture over top. Serves 4.

1 serving: 273 Calories; 7.5 g Total Fat (2.0 g Mono, 0.3 g Poly, 4.5 g Sat); 19 mg Cholesterol; 54 g Carbohydrate; 2 g Fibre; 2 g Protein; 81 mg Sodium

Hot Fudge Mondaes

Make your Mondays a little bit brighter with this low-fat alternative to a hot fudge sundae! Substitute your favourite fruit for the strawberries on Tuesday, Wednesday, Thursday...

HOT FUDGE SAUCE

Granulated sugar	3/4 cup	175 mL
Cocoa, sifted if lumpy	1/4 cup	60 mL
Cornstarch	2 tbsp.	30 mL
Skim evaporated milk	1/2 cup	125 mL
Vanilla extract	1 tsp.	5 mL

SUNDAES

Non-fat vanilla frozen yogurt	2 cups	500 mL
Sliced fresh strawberries	1 cup	250 mL

Hot Fudge Sauce: Combine first 4 ingredients in small heavy saucepan. Heat and stir on medium until boiling and thickened. Remove from heat.

Add vanilla. Stir. Let stand, uncovered, for 15 minutes. Makes about 1 cup (250 mL) sauce.

Sundaes: Spoon frozen yogurt into 4 small bowls. Drizzle with Hot Fudge Sauce. Top with strawberries. Serves 4.

1 serving: 304 Calories; 1.0 g Total Fat (0.3 g Mono, 0.1 g Poly, 0.6 g Sat); 3 mg Cholesterol; 68 g Carbohydrate; 2 g Fibre; 8 g Protein; 103 mg Sodium

Pictured on page 107.

Maple Bourbon Pears

Sophisticated in taste but easy to prepare, these bourbon-soaked pears are magnificent with a dollop of light whipped topping, or a scoop of vanilla frozen yogurt.

Maple (or maple-flavoured) syrup	1/2 cup	125 mL
Bourbon whiskey	1/4 cup	60 mL
Brown sugar, packed	1 tbsp.	15 mL
Ground cinnamon	1/4 tsp.	1 mL
Ground cloves, sprinkle		
Large peeled pears, cored and quartered	4	4

Preheat oven to 450°F (230°C). Combine first 5 ingredients in small bowl.

Place pears, cut-side up, in greased 2 quart (2 L) shallow baking dish. Pour maple mixture over top. Bake for about 20 minutes, spooning sauce over pears at halftime, until pears are tender and edges are golden. Serves 4.

1 serving: 270 Calories; 0.3 g Total Fat (0.1 g Mono, 0.1 g Poly, trace Sat); 0 mg Cholesterol; 62 g Carbohydrate; 7 g Fibre; 1 g Protein; 7 mg Sodium

Pictured on page 143.

Mango Rhubarb Fool

Don't be fooled by the title—this is a low-fat version of the rich dessert commonly made with fruit and whipped cream.

Chopped frozen rhubarb	3 cups	750 mL
Granulated sugar	1 cup	250 mL
Can of sliced mango in syrup, drained and chopped	14 oz.	398 mL
Low-fat plain yogurt	2 cups	500 mL
Medium sweetened coconut, toasted (see Tip, page 149), optional	4 tsp.	20 mL

(continued on next page)

Combine rhubarb and sugar in medium saucepan. Cook, uncovered, on medium for about 10 minutes, stirring occasionally, until rhubarb is tender. Transfer to medium bowl. Carefully place medium bowl in large bowl, filled halfway with ice water. Let stand for about 8 minutes, stirring often, until cool.

Add mango. Stir. Add yogurt. Stir well. Spoon into 6 dessert bowls.

Sprinkle coconut over top. Makes about 4 1/2 cups (1.1 L). Serves 6.

1 serving: 240 Calories; 1.1 g Total Fat (0 g Mono, 0 g Poly, 0.8 g Sat); 7 mg Cholesterol; 55 g Carbohydrate; 2 g Fibre; 4 g Protein; 60 mg Sodium

Stewed Fruit Sundaes

Healthy dried fruit with sweet cinnamon and delicate anise is the perfect topper for frozen yogurt. For a breakfast treat, spoon it over yogurt or oatmeal.

STEWED FRUIT		
Diced unpeeled pear	1 cup	250 mL
Water	1 cup	250 mL
Halved dried apricots	1/2 cup	125 mL
Raisins	1/4 cup	60 mL
Grated orange zest	2 tsp.	10 mL
Cinnamon stick (4 inches, 10 cm)	1	1
Star anise (optional)	1	1
SUNDAES		
Non-fat vanilla frozen yogurt	2 cups	500 mL

Stewed Fruit: Combine all 7 ingredients in medium saucepan. Bring to a boil. Reduce heat to medium. Boil gently, uncovered, for about 15 minutes, stirring occasionally, until fruit is tender and mixture is slightly syrupy. Remove and discard cinnamon stick and anise. Makes about 1 1/3 cups (325 mL) fruit.

Sundaes: Spoon frozen yogurt into 4 small bowls. Spoon Stewed Fruit over top. Serves 4.

1 serving: 203 Calories; 0.3 g Total Fat (0.1 g Mono, trace Poly, 0.1 g Sat); 2 mg Cholesterol; 47 g Carbohydrate; 4 g Fibre; 6 g Protein; 78 mg Sodium

Grilled Peaches

Fire up the grill for this delectable delicacy. The balsamic vinegar and honey caramelize to form a tangy and sweet coating on the warm, tender peaches.

Balsamic vinegar	1/4 cup	60 mL
Liquid honey	2 tbsp.	30 mL
Olive (or canola) oil	2 tsp.	10 mL
Finely chopped fresh mint	1 tbsp.	15 mL
(or 3/4 tsp., 4 mL, dried)		
Fresh peaches, halved	4	4
(or 8 canned peach halves)		
Frozen whipped topping, thawed (optional)	1/2 cup	125 mL

Preheat gas barbecue to medium-high. Whisk first 3 ingredients in large bowl. Add mint. Stir.

Add peaches. Toss until coated. Place peaches, cut-side down, on greased grill. Close lid. Cook for 6 to 8 minutes, turning once and brushing with vinegar mixture, until peaches are tender but still hold their shape. Place peaches on 4 dessert plates.

Spoon whipped topping over peaches. Serves 4.

1 serving: 125 Calories; 2.6 g Total Fat (1.8 g Mono, 0.3 g Poly, 0.3 g Sat); 0 mg Cholesterol; 26 g Carbohydrate; 2 g Fibre; 1 g Protein; 5 mg Sodium

Chocolate Pudding

Forgo those store-bought low-fat puddings full of chemicals. This rich pudding with a dark chocolate flavour is all natural. Best served warm.

Granulated sugar	1/2 cup	125 mL
Cocoa, sifted if lumpy	1/4 cup	60 mL
Cornstarch	1/4 cup	60 mL
Salt	1/8 tsp.	0.5 mL
Skim milk	2 1/2 cups	625 mL
Semi-sweet chocolate baking squares	2	2
(1 oz., 28 g, each), coarsely chopped		
Vanilla extract	1 1/2 tsp.	7 mL

(continued on next page)

Combine first 4 ingredients in medium heavy saucepan. Stir in milk. Bring to a boil on medium, stirring constantly. Heat and stir until boiling and thickened. Remove from heat.

Add chocolate and vanilla. Stir until chocolate is melted. Spoon into 4 small bowls. Makes about 2 2/3 cups (650 mL). Serves 4.

1 serving: 264 Calories; 5.0 g Total Fat (0.3 g Mono, trace Poly, 3.1 g Sat); 3 mg Cholesterol; 51 g Carbohydrate; 2 g Fibre; 7 g Protein; 154 mg Sodium

Broiled Pineapple

This perfectly pleasing pineapple is quick and easy to make when you use the ready-to-eat, peeled and cored fresh pineapples available in most supermarkets. Serve warm with light whipped topping.

Fresh pineapple slices (1inch, 2.5 cm, thick), cores removed	4	4
Orange marmalade	1/4 cup	60 mL
Lemon juice	1 tsp.	5 mL
Minced crystallized ginger	1/2 tsp.	2 mL
Granulated sugar	2 tsp.	10 mL
Ground cinnamon	1/8 tsp.	0.5 mL

Preheat broiler. Arrange pineapple slices on baking sheet with sides, lined with greased foil.

Combine next 3 ingredients in small saucepan. Heat and stir on medium until marmalade is melted. Brush over pineapple. Broil on top rack in oven for about 5 minutes until golden and bubbling.

Combine sugar and cinnamon in small cup. Sprinkle over pineapple. Serves 2.

1 serving: 173 Calories; 0.1 g Total Fat (trace Mono, 0.1 g Poly, trace Sat); 0 mg Cholesterol; 46 g Carbohydrate; 2 g Fibre; 1 g Protein; 24 mg Sodium

Pictured on page 126.

Rhubarb Ginger Sundaes

For a tart and gingery treat, a tasty rhubarb compote
can't be beat. Served over frozen yogurt with flair,
you won't find a healthier dessert anywhere.

RHUBARB GINGER SAUCE

Chopped fresh (or frozen) rhubarb	5 cups	1.25 L
Brown sugar, packed	3/4 cup	175 mL
Gingerroot slices (1/4 inch, 6 mm, thick)	4	4
Minced crystallized ginger	2 tbsp.	30 mL
Orange liqueur	1 tbsp.	15 mL
Grated orange zest	1 tsp.	5 mL

SUNDAES

Non-fat vanilla frozen yogurt	6 cups	1.5 L

Rhubarb Ginger Sauce: Combine first 4 ingredients in large saucepan. Cover. Bring to a boil on medium. Reduce heat to medium-low. Simmer for about 10 minutes until rhubarb is soft. Remove and discard gingerroot.

Stir in liqueur and orange zest. Makes about 2 2/3 cups (650 mL) sauce.

Sundaes: Spoon frozen yogurt into 6 small bowls. Spoon rhubarb mixture over top. Serves 6.

1 serving: 340 Calories; 0.5 g Total Fat (0.1 g Mono, 0.1 g Poly, 0.3 g Sat); 3 mg Cholesterol; 75 g Carbohydrate; 2 g Fibre; 11 g Protein; 147 mg Sodium

BLUBARB SUNDAES: Reduce rhubarb to 3 cups (750 mL). Add 2 cups (500 mL) fresh (or frozen) blueberries.

STRAWBARB SUNDAES: Reduce rhubarb to 3 cups (750 mL). Add 2 cups (500 mL) fresh (or frozen) strawberries.

BUMBLEBARB SUNDAES: Reduce rhubarb to 3 cups (750 mL). Add 2 cups (500 mL) fresh (or frozen) mixed berries.

Desserts

Spiced Clusters

A perfect blend of sugar and spice, these healthy clusters
are low-fat and sure to please the most finicky snack fiend.

Butter (or hard margarine), softened	1/3 cup	75 mL
Brown sugar, packed	2/3 cup	150 mL
Egg whites (large)	2	2
Unsweetened applesauce	1/2 cup	125 mL
Quick-cooking rolled oats	1 1/2 cups	375 mL
Whole-wheat flour	1/4 cup	60 mL
Ground flaxseed	2 tbsp.	30 mL
Sesame seeds	2 tbsp.	30 mL
Ground cinnamon	1 tsp.	5 mL
Baking powder	1/2 tsp.	2 mL
Ground ginger	1/2 tsp.	2 mL
Ground allspice	1/8 tsp.	0.5 mL
Chopped pitted dates	1/4 cup	60 mL
Dried cranberries	1/4 cup	60 mL
Sliced natural almonds	1/4 cup	60 mL
Grated lemon zest	1 tsp.	5 mL

Preheat oven to 375°F (190°C). Cream butter and brown sugar in large bowl. Add egg whites, 1 at a time, mixing well after each addition. Stir in applesauce.

Combine next 8 ingredients in medium bowl. Add to butter mixture. Mix until no dry flour remains.

Add remaining 4 ingredients. Mix well. Drop, using about 1 tbsp. (15 mL) for each, about 2 inches (5 cm) apart onto greased cookie sheets. Press lightly with fork to flatten. Bake on separate racks in oven for 8 to 10 minutes, switching position of cookie sheets at halftime, until golden. Let stand on cookie sheets for 5 minutes. Remove clusters from cookie sheets and place on wire racks to cool. Makes about 30 clusters.

1 cluster: 78 Calories; 3.3 g Total Fat (1.0 g Mono, 0.4 g Poly, 1.4 g Sat); 5 mg Cholesterol; 11 g Carbohydrate; 1 g Fibre; 2 g Protein; 24 mg Sodium

Pictured on page 144.

Cranberry Applesauce Cookies

They'll be stepping up to the plate to grab a couple of these satisfying treats.

Quick-cooking rolled oats	1 cup	250 mL
All-purpose flour	3/4 cup	175 mL
Baking powder	1/2 tsp.	2 mL
Baking soda	1/4 tsp.	1 mL
Salt	1/4 tsp.	1 mL
Large egg	1	1
Brown sugar, packed	1/4 cup	60 mL
Granulated sugar	1/4 cup	60 mL
Unsweetened applesauce	1/4 cup	60 mL
Butter (or hard margarine), melted	2 tbsp.	30 mL
Vanilla extract	1/2 tsp.	2 mL
Dried cranberries	1/4 cup	60 mL

Preheat oven to 375°F (190°C). Combine first 5 ingredients in medium bowl. Set aside.

Beat next 6 ingredients in large bowl until smooth and creamy.

Add cranberries and flour mixture. Stir well. Spray large cookie sheet with cooking spray. Drop, using about 1 tbsp. (15 mL) for each, about 1 inch (2.5 cm) apart onto cookie sheet. Bake for about 10 minutes until golden. Let stand on cookie sheet for 5 minutes. Remove cookies from cookie sheet and place on wire rack to cool. Makes about 18 cookies.

1 cookie: 79 Calories; 1.9 g Total Fat (0.5 g Mono, 0.1 g Poly, 0.9 g Sat); 14 mg Cholesterol; 14 g Carbohydrate; 1 g Fibre; 2 g Protein; 71 mg Sodium

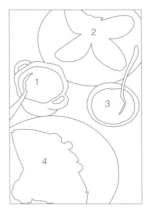

1. Hot Pudding Cakes, page 129
2. Maple Bourbon Pears, page 136
3. Blueberry Peach Crumble, page 131
4. Chocolate Crepes, page 130

Props courtesy of: Danesco Inc.
　　　　　　　　　Mikasa Home Store

Snacks

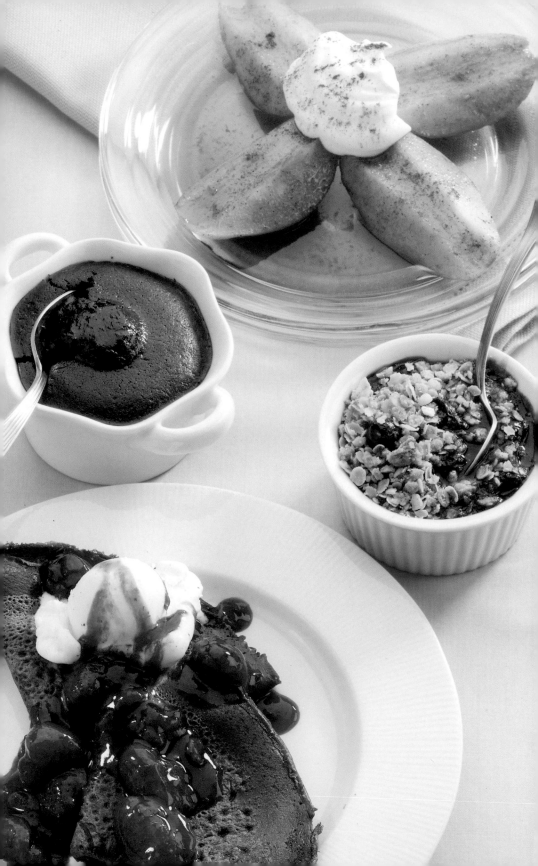

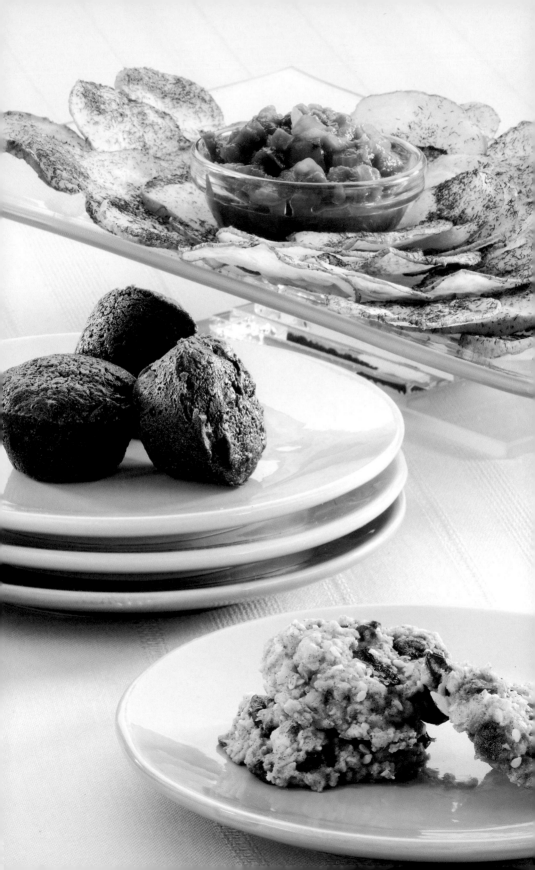

Dill-icious Potato Chips

Yes, there is room in a low-fat cookbook for this favourite, salty snack. Baked to perfection, try dipping these in non-fat sour cream, salsa or fat-free dressing.

Unpeeled potatoes	1 lb.	454 g
Cooking spray		
Dried dillweed	1 1/2 tsp.	7 mL
Seasoned salt	1 1/2 tsp.	7 mL

Preheat oven to 450°F (230°C). Cut potatoes crosswise into 1/8 inch (3 mm) thick slices.

Arrange potato slices in single layer on 2 greased baking sheets with sides. Spray with cooking spray. Sprinkle dill and seasoned salt over top. Bake on separate racks in oven for 15 to 20 minutes, switching position of baking sheets at halftime, removing chips from baking sheets as they become brown and crisp around edges. Makes about 36 chips. Serves 2.

1 serving: 173 Calories; 0.3 g Total Fat (trace Mono, 0.1 g Poly, 0.1 g Sat); 0 mg Cholesterol; 39 g Carbohydrate; 4 g Fibre; 5 g Protein; 1070 mg Sodium

Pictured at left.

TACO POTATO CHIPS: Instead of dillweed and seasoned salt, use 1 tbsp. (15 mL) taco seasoning.

BARBECUE STEAK POTATO CHIPS: Instead of dillweed and seasoned salt, use 1 tbsp. (15 mL) Montreal steak spice.

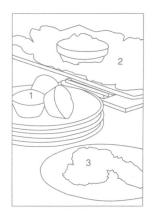

1. Guilt-Free Mini Brownies, page 146
2. Dill-icious Potato Chips, above
3. Spiced Clusters, page 141

Props courtesy of: Winners Stores

Snacks

Curry Pretzels

Turn a favourite nibble into a sweet, savoury treat. Curry powder and honey turn pretzels into snack heaven. These are definitely "knot" ordinary!

Small pretzels	4 cups	1 L
Liquid honey	3 tbsp.	50 mL
Butter (or hard margarine)	2 tsp.	10 mL
Curry powder	1 1/2 tsp.	7 mL

Preheat oven to 350°F (175°C). Put pretzels into large bowl.

Combine remaining 3 ingredients in small microwave-safe bowl. Microwave, uncovered, on high (100%) for about 60 seconds until hot and bubbling. Stir. Pour over pretzels. Toss until coated. Arrange on greased large baking sheet with sides. Bake for 10 minutes, stirring at halftime. Transfer pretzels to large plate to cool. Stir gently to separate. Makes about 4 cups (1 L). Serves 8.

1 serving: 99 Calories; 1.6 g Total Fat (0.5 g Mono, 0.3 g Poly, 0.7 g Sat); 3 mg Cholesterol; 20 g Carbohydrate; 1 g Fibre; 2 g Protein; 296 mg Sodium

Guilt-Free Mini Brownies

Brownies without the guilt? Oh, yeah! These chewy, chocolatey bites will satisfy your sweet tooth in a second.

Semi-sweet chocolate baking squares (1 oz., 28 g, each), coarsely chopped	2	2
Granulated sugar	1 cup	250 mL
All-purpose flour	2/3 cup	150 mL
Cocoa, sifted if lumpy	1/2 cup	125 mL
Salt	1/4 tsp.	1 mL
Large egg	1	1
Egg whites (large)	2	2
Whole cranberry sauce	1/2 cup	125 mL
Canola oil	2 tbsp.	30 mL

(continued on next page)

Preheat oven to 350°F (175°C). Put chocolate into small microwave-safe bowl. Microwave, uncovered, on medium (50%) for about 90 seconds, stirring every 30 seconds, until almost melted (see Tip, page 129). Do not overheat. Stir until smooth.

Meanwhile, measure next 4 ingredients into medium bowl. Stir. Make a well in centre.

Whisk remaining 4 ingredients and melted chocolate in small bowl until combined. Add to well. Stir until just moistened. Fill 24 greased mini-muffin cups 3/4 full. Bake for about 15 minutes until wooden pick inserted in centre of brownie comes out moist but not wet with batter. Do not overbake. Makes 24 mini-brownies.

1 mini-brownie: 81 Calories; 2.2 g Total Fat (0.8 g Mono, 0.4 g Poly, 0.7 g Sat); 8 mg Cholesterol; 15 g Carbohydrate; 1 g Fibre; 1 g Protein; 34 mg Sodium

Pictured on page 144.

Pesto Popcorn

Popcorn is dressed in pesto, and presto—a crunchy favourite gets a magical makeover!

Bag of trans fat-free microwave popcorn	3 oz.	80 g
Grated light Parmesan cheese	2 tbsp.	30 mL
Dried basil	1 tsp.	5 mL
Parsley flakes	1/2 tsp.	2 mL
Garlic powder	1/4 tsp.	1 mL
Cooking spray		

Microwave popcorn on high (100%) for 2 to 3 minutes until popping slows to 1 second between pops. Carefully remove bag from microwave. Transfer popcorn to extra-large bowl.

Combine next 4 ingredients in small cup.

Spray popcorn with cooking spray for 2 to 3 seconds. Sprinkle with half of cheese mixture. Toss until coated. Spray with cooking spray for another 2 to 3 seconds. Sprinkle with remaining cheese mixture. Toss until coated. Makes about 12 cups (3 L). Serves 4.

1 serving: 121 Calories; 3.5 g Total Fat (0.9 g Mono, 0.8 g Poly, 0.3 g Sat); 7 mg Cholesterol; 19 g Carbohydrate; 3 g Fibre; 4 g Protein; 211 mg Sodium

Apricot Macaroons

Grab a cup of coffee or tea and treat yourself to these marvellous macaroons.
Loads of sweetness without all the fat. Guilt-free snacking at its best!

Egg whites (large)	2	2
Icing (confectioner's) sugar	1 cup	250 mL
Medium unsweetened coconut	1 1/2 cups	375 mL
Chopped dried apricot	1 cup	250 mL

Preheat oven to 350°F (175°C). Whisk egg whites in large bowl until frothy. Add icing sugar. Stir until smooth.

Add coconut and apricot. Stir well. Drop, using about 1 tbsp. (15 mL) for each, onto 2 parchment (not waxed) paper-lined cookie sheets. Bake on separate racks in oven for about 12 minutes, switching position of cookie sheets at halftime, until golden. Let stand on cookie sheets for 5 minutes. Remove macaroons from cookie sheets and place on wire rack to cool. Makes about 24 macaroons.

1 macaroon: 65 Calories; 3.0 g Total Fat (0.1 g Mono, trace Poly, 2.7 g Sat); 0 mg Cholesterol; 10 g Carbohydrate; 1 g Fibre; 1 g Protein; 10 mg Sodium

Apple Cheddar Bagels

The ages-old marriage of apple and Cheddar renews its vows
in a new setting—a crisp bagel topped with cinnamon sugar.

Whole-grain (or whole-wheat) bagels, split	2	2
Thinly sliced unpeeled apple	1 cup	250 mL
Brown sugar, packed	1 tbsp.	15 mL
Ground cinnamon	1/2 tsp.	2 mL
Grated light sharp Cheddar cheese	1/2 cup	125 mL

Preheat oven to 350°F (175°C). Toast bagel halves. Place, cut-side up, on ungreased baking sheet.

Put apple into small bowl. Sprinkle with brown sugar and cinnamon. Toss until coated. Arrange on bagel halves.

(continued on next page)

Sprinkle with cheese. Bake for about 10 minutes until apple is tender. Cut into 2 pieces each. Serves 4.

1 serving: 170 Calories; 5.7 g Total Fat (1.3 g Mono, 1.2 g Poly, 3.0 g Sat); 15 mg Cholesterol; 26 g Carbohydrate; 4 g Fibre; 7 g Protein; 189 mg Sodium

Fruit And Nut Bites

Looking for an energy boost and a treat all rolled into one? Then these fruity, nutty bites are right up your alley. They're sure to bowl over family and friends.

Orange juice	1/2 cup	125 mL
Dried apricots	1 1/2 cups	375 mL
Raisins	1/2 cup	125 mL
Dried pitted prunes	1/4 cup	60 mL
Ground almonds, toasted (see Tip, below)	1/2 cup	125 mL
Fine coconut	1/2 cup	125 mL

Measure orange juice into small saucepan. Bring to a boil. Reduce heat to medium-low. Add next 3 ingredients. Simmer, uncovered, for about 5 minutes until fruit is plump. Drain, reserving 1 tbsp. (15 mL) cooking liquid. Transfer fruit and reserved cooking liquid to food processor. Process with on/off motion for about 1 minute until finely chopped. Transfer to small bowl.

Add almonds. Stir well. Let stand for 2 to 3 minutes until cool enough to handle. Roll into 1 inch (2.5 cm) balls.

Spread coconut on large plate. Roll balls in coconut until coated. Makes about 28 bites.

1 bite: 54 Calories; 1.9 g Total Fat (0.6 g Mono, 0.2 g Poly, 1.0 g Sat); 0 mg Cholesterol; 9 g Carbohydrate; 1 g Fibre; 1 g Protein; 6 mg Sodium

 tip When toasting nuts, seeds or coconut, cooking times will vary for each type of nut—so never toast them together. For small amounts, place ingredient in an ungreased shallow frying pan. Heat on medium for 3 to 5 minutes, stirring often, until golden. For larger amounts, spread ingredient evenly in an ungreased shallow pan. Bake in a 350°F (175°C) oven for 5 to 10 minutes, stirring or shaking often, until golden.

Measurement Tables

Throughout this book measurements are given in Conventional and Metric measure. To compensate for differences between the two measurements due to rounding, a full metric measure is not always used. The cup used is the standard 8 fluid ounce. Temperature is given in degrees Fahrenheit and Celsius. Baking pan measurements are in inches and centimetres as well as quarts and litres. An exact metric conversion is given below as well as the working equivalent (Metric Standard Measure).

Spoons

Conventional Measure	Metric Exact Conversion Millilitre (mL)	Metric Standard Measure Millilitre (mL)
1/8 teaspoon (tsp.)	0.6 mL	0.5 mL
1/4 teaspoon (tsp.)	1.2 mL	1 mL
1/2 teaspoon (tsp.)	2.4 mL	2 mL
1 teaspoon (tsp.)	4.7 mL	5 mL
2 teaspoons (tsp.)	9.4 mL	10 mL
1 tablespoon (tbsp.)	14.2 mL	15 mL

Cups

Conventional Measure	Metric Exact Conversion Millilitre (mL)	Metric Standard Measure Millilitre (mL)
1/4 cup (4 tbsp.)	56.8 mL	60 mL
1/3 cup (5 1/3 tbsp.)	75.6 mL	75 mL
1/2 cup (8 tbsp.)	113.7 mL	125 mL
2/3 cup (10 2/3 tbsp.)	151.2 mL	150 mL
3/4 cup (12 tbsp.)	170.5 mL	175 mL
1 cup (16 tbsp.)	227.3 mL	250 mL
4 1/2 cups	1022.9 mL	1000 mL (1 L)

Oven Temperatures

Fahrenheit (°F)	Celsius (°C)
175°	80°
200°	95°
225°	110°
250°	120°
275°	140°
300°	150°
325°	160°
350°	175°
375°	190°
400°	205°
425°	220°
450°	230°
475°	240°
500°	260°

Dry Measurements

Conventional Measure Ounces (oz.)	Metric Exact Conversion Grams (g)	Metric Standard Measure Grams (g)
1 oz.	28.3 g	28 g
2 oz.	56.7 g	57 g
3 oz.	85.0 g	85 g
4 oz.	113.4 g	125 g
5 oz.	141.7 g	140 g
6 oz.	170.1 g	170 g
7 oz.	198.4 g	200 g
8 oz.	226.8 g	250 g
16 oz.	453.6 g	500 g
32 oz.	907.2 g	1000 g (1 kg)

Pans

Conventional Inches	Metric Centimetres
8x8 inch	20x20 cm
9x9 inch	22x22 cm
9x13 inch	22x33 cm
10x15 inch	25x38 cm
11x17 inch	28x43 cm
8x2 inch round	20x5 cm
9x2 inch round	22x5 cm
10x4 1/2 inch tube	25x11 cm
8x4x3 inch loaf	20x10x7.5 cm
9x5x3 inch loaf	22x12.5x7.5 cm

Casseroles

CANADA & BRITAIN		UNITED STATES	
Standard Size Casserole	Exact Metric Measure	Standard Size Casserole	Exact Metric Measure
1 qt. (5 cups)	1.13 L	1 qt. (4 cups)	900 mL
1 1/2 qts. (7 1/2 cups)	1.69 L	1 1/2 qts. (6 cups)	1.35 L
2 qts. (10 cups)	2.25 L	2 qts. (8 cups)	1.8 L
2 1/2 qts. (12 1/2 cups)	2.81 L	2 1/2 qts. (10 cups)	2.25 L
3 qts. (15 cups)	3.38 L	3 qts. (12 cups)	2.7 L
4 qts. (20 cups)	4.5 L	4 qts. (16 cups)	3.6 L
5 qts. (25 cups)	5.63 L	5 qts. (20 cups)	4.5 L

Recipe Index

E

F

G

H

J

L

153

154

155

Company's Coming cookbooks are available at retail locations throughout Canada!

EXCLUSIVE mail order offer on next page

Buy any 2 cookbooks—choose a 3rd FREE of equal or lesser value than the lowest price paid.

Original Series — CA$15.99 Canada — US$12.99 USA & International

CODE		CODE		CODE	
SQ	150 Delicious Squares	PB	The Potato Book	WM	30-Minute Weekday Meals
CA	Casseroles	CCLFC	Low-Fat Cooking	SDL	School Days Lunches
MU	Muffins & More	SCH	Stews, Chilies & Chowders	PD	Potluck Dishes
SA	Salads	FD	Fondues	GBR	Ground Beef Recipes
AP	Appetizers	CCBE	The Beef Book	FRIR	4-Ingredient Recipes
CO	Cookies	RC	The Rookie Cook	KHC	Kids' Healthy Cooking
PA	Pasta	RHR	Rush-Hour Recipes	MM	Mostly Muffins
BA	Barbecues	SW	Sweet Cravings	SP	Soups
PR	Preserves	YRG	Year-Round Grilling	SU	Simple Suppers
CH	Chicken, Etc.	GG	Garden Greens	CCDC	Diabetic Cooking
CT	Cooking For Two	CHC	Chinese Cooking	CHN	Chicken Now
SC	Slow Cooker Recipes	RL	Recipes For Leftovers	KDS	Kids Do Snacks
SF	Stir-Fry	BEV	The Beverage Book	TMRC	30-Minute Rookie Cook
MAM	Make-Ahead Meals	SCD	Slow Cooker Dinners		

Cookbook Author Biography

CODE	CA$15.99 Canada US$12.99 USA & International
JP	Jean Paré: An Appetite for Life

Most Loved Recipe Collection

CODE	CA$23.99 Canada US$19.99 USA & International
MLBQ	Most Loved Barbecuing
MLCO	Most Loved Cookies

CODE	CA$24.99 Canada US$19.99 USA & International
MLSD	Most Loved Salads & Dressings
MLCA	Most Loved Casseroles
MLSF	Most Loved Stir-Fries
MLHF	Most Loved Holiday Favourites

3-in-1 Cookbook Collection

CODE	CA$29.99 Canada US$24.99 USA & International
MNT	Meals in No Time

Lifestyle Series

CODE	CA$17.99 Canada US$15.99 USA & International
DC	Diabetic Cooking

CODE	CA$19.99 Canada US$15.99 USA & International
DDI	Diabetic Dinners
HR	Easy Healthy Recipes
HH	Healthy in a Hurry
WGR	Whole Grain Recipes

Special Occasion Series

CODE	CA$20.99 Canada US$19.99 USA & International
GFK	Gifts from the Kitchen

CODE	CA$24.99 Canada US$19.99 USA & International
MLBQ	Christmas Gifts from the Kitchen
TR	Timeless Recipes for All Occasions

CODE	CA$27.99 Canada US$22.99 USA & International
CCEL	Christmas Celebrations

CODE	CA$29.99 Canada US$24.99 USA & International
CATH	Cooking At Home

Order **ONLINE** for fast delivery!

Log onto **www.companyscoming.com**, browse through our library of cookbooks, gift sets and newest releases and place your order using our fast and secure online order form.

Buy 2, Get 1 FREE!

Buy any 2 cookbooks—choose a **3rd FREE** of equal or lesser value than the lowest price paid.

Title	Code	Quantity	Price	Total
			$	$
DON'T FORGET to indicate your FREE BOOK(S). (see exclusive mail order offer above) please print				

		TOTAL BOOKS (including FREE)		TOTAL BOOKS PURCHASED:	

	International	USA	Canada
Shipping & Handling First Book (per destination)	$ 11.98 (one book)	$ 6.98 (one book)	$ 5.98 (one book)
Additional Books (include FREE books)	$ ($4.99 each)	$ ($1.99 each)	$ ($1.99 each)
Sub-Total	$	$	$
Canadian residents add GST/HST			$
TOTAL AMOUNT ENCLOSED	$	$	$

Terms

- All orders must be prepaid. Sorry, no CODs.
- Prices are listed in Canadian Funds for Canadian orders, or US funds for US & International orders.
- Prices are subject to change without prior notice.
- Canadian residents must pay GST/HST (no provincial tax required).
- No tax is required for orders outside Canada.
- Satisfaction is guaranteed or return within 30 days for a full refund.
- Make cheque or money order payable to: **Company's Coming Publishing Limited** 2311-96 Street, Edmonton, Alberta Canada T6N 1G3.
- Orders are shipped surface mail. For courier rates, visit our website: **www.companyscoming.com** or contact us: **Tel: 780-450-6223 Fax: 780-450-1857.**

Gift Giving

- Let us help you with your gift giving!
- We will send cookbooks directly to the recipients of your choice if you give us their names and addresses.
- Please specify the titles you wish to send to each person.
- If you would like to include a personal note or card, we will be pleased to enclose it with your gift order.
- Company's Coming Cookbooks make excellent gifts: birthdays, bridal showers, Mother's Day, Father's Day, graduation or any occasion …collect them all!

☐ MasterCard   ☐ VISA   Expiry ____ / ____ MO/YR

Credit Card # _____

Name of cardholder _____

Cardholder signature _____

Shipping Address Send the cookbooks listed above to:

☐ **Please check if this is a Gift Order**

Name: _____

Street: _____

City: _____ Prov./State: _____

Postal Code/Zip: _____ Country: _____

Tel: (____) _____

E-mail address: _____

Your privacy is important to us. We will not share your e-mail address or personal information with any outside party.

☐ **YES! Please add me to your News Bite e-mail newsletter.**

Cookmark

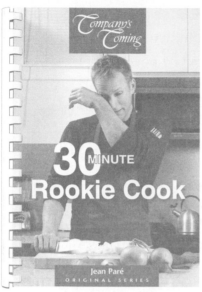

Does the thought of creating fast, fabulous meals bring fear to your heart and tears to your eyes? With over 130 speedy and trouble-free recipes, *30-Minute Rookie Cook*—a sequel to our best-selling *Rookie Cook*—is your key to easy home cooking in a half hour or less!

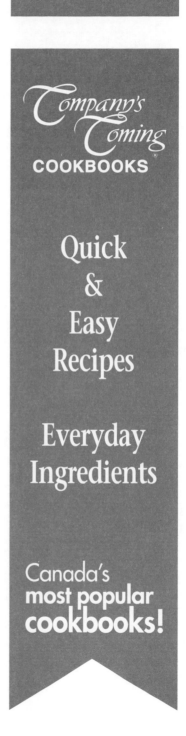

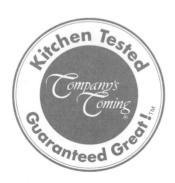

Complete your Original Series Collection!

- ❏ 150 Delicious Squares
- ❏ Casseroles
- ❏ Muffins & More
- ❏ Salads
- ❏ Appetizers
- ❏ Cookies
- ❏ Pasta
- ❏ Barbecues
- ❏ Preserves
- ❏ Chicken, Etc.
- ❏ Cooking For Two
- ❏ Slow Cooker Recipes
- ❏ Stir-Fry
- ❏ Make-Ahead Meals
- ❏ The Potato Book
- ❏ Low-Fat Cooking
- ❏ Stews, Chilies & Chowders
- ❏ Fondues
- ❏ The Beef Book
- ❏ The Rookie Cook
- ❏ Rush-Hour Recipes
- ❏ Sweet Cravings
- ❏ Year-Round Grilling
- ❏ Garden Greens
- ❏ Chinese Cooking
- ❏ Recipes For Leftovers
- ❏ The Beverage Book
- ❏ Slow Cooker Dinners
- ❏ 30-Minute Weekday Meals
- ❏ School Days Lunches
- ❏ Potluck Dishes
- ❏ Ground Beef Recipes
- ❏ 4-Ingredient Recipes
- ❏ Kids' Healthy Cooking
- ❏ Mostly Muffins
- ❏ Soups
- ❏ Simple Suppers
- ❏ Diabetic Cooking
- ❏ Chicken Now
- ❏ Kids Do Snacks
- ❏ 30-Minute Rookie Cook

FREE Online NEWSLETTER

- **FREE** recipes & cooking tips
- **Exclusive** cookbook offers
- **Preview** new titles

Subscribe today!

www.companyscoming.com

COLLECT ALL Company's Coming Series Cookbooks!

Most Loved Recipe Collection

- ❏ Most Loved Barbecuing
- ❏ Most Loved Cookies
- ❏ Most Loved Salads & Dressings
- ❏ Most Loved Casseroles
- ❏ Most Loved Stir-Fries
- ❏ Most Loved Holiday Favourites

Lifestyle Series

- ❏ Diabetic Cooking
- ❏ Diabetic Dinners
- ❏ Easy Healthy Recipes
- ❏ Whole Grain Recipes

Special Occasion Series

- ❏ Gifts from the Kitchen
- ❏ Christmas Gifts from the Kitchen
- ❏ Timeless Recipes for All Occasions
- ❏ Christmas Celebrations
- ❏ Cooking at Home

Cookbook Author Biography

- ❏ Jean Paré: An Appetite for Life

3-in-1 Cookbook Collection

- ❏ Meals in No Time

Canada's most popular cookbooks!